Living Well Naturally

Also by Anthony J. Sattilaro, M.D.
with Tom Monte

Recalled by Life:
The Story of My Recovery from Cancer

Living Well Naturally

Anthony J. Sattilaro, M.D.
and Tom Monte

Boston
HOUGHTON MIFFLIN COMPANY

The appendix appears with the permission of the
Center for Science in the Public Interest.

Library of Congress Cataloging in Publication Data

Sattilaro, Anthony J.
Living well naturally.

Bibliography: p.
1. Nutrition. 2. Health. 3. Nutritionally induced
diseases. 4. Cancer—Nutritional aspects. 5. Sattilaro,
Anthony J. 6. Cancer—Patients—United States—
Biography. I. Monte, Tom. II. Title.
RA784.S36 1984   613   83-22623
ISBN 0-395-34422-0

Printed in the United States of America

S 10 9 8 7 6 5 4 3 2

To the Lamb of God,
Who takes away the sin of the world
and grants us peace

For now we see through a glass, darkly; but then face to face; now I know in part; but then shall I know even as also I am known.

I COR. 13:12

We would like to express our deep gratitude to A. Grant Sprecher, Esquire, for his review of the manuscript and to Helga Newmark for writing and testing all the recipes provided in this book.

Contents

Preface *ix*

PART I

1. A Change in Lifestyle *1*
2. Your Diet and Health *10*
3. Your New Healthy Diet *43*
4. Your New Exercise Program *82*
5. How the Mind Affects the Body *96*
6. The Power of Faith *107*
7. Exercises for Peace of Mind *135*
8. A Program for Good Health *148*

    Hope, Faith, and Love *161*

PART II

9. Cooking for Life *165*
10. The Recipes *174*
    Whole Grains *174*
    Vegetables *185*
    Beans *191*
    Seaweeds *199*
    Animal Foods *200*
    Condiments and Dressings *202*
    Fruits and Desserts *204*

Appendix: Fat and Calorie Content
of Selected Foods   *211*
Bibliography   220

Preface

THE APPARENTLY happy ending of my first book, *Recalled by Life,* has me leaving the peaceful silence of the Cathedral of Peter and Paul and walking into the sunlight of an exciting Philadelphia day. But what has happened since? Has the sunlight continued? Have the cancer and all the evil that created and nurtured it been slain forever? These hopes are what we dream about — but we know deep inside that in reality sunlight must be interrupted with shadows of doubt and struggle.

I remain physically strong, almost vibrantly healthy — what some might call "born again." Yet that is not the end of the story; for if it were, this strange diet, coupled with man's enormous genius in science, would have conquered all our ills generations ago. The diet helped me to become strong in body, "centered" if you will, but then it opened a whole new realm of spiritual challenges that my rational self could never before have imagined. But to say that diet alone cured me would be to have me fall into the magic bullet trap that has consistently ensnared all of us as we reach for paradise on earth.

As my body expelled the cancer and the many other poisons that had been produced over the years of self-indulgence, my euphoria of victory passed, and once again, though physically well, I felt the inner loneliness that none of us can escape, even at the height of success. I began to realize that the now cleansed body was crying out for spiritual nourishment — crying out to the same Spirit that had given it such perfection at birth only to be destroyed by my inward turning as I grew. The diet alone could not have sustained me; I had to grow on the love that had created me fifty-two years ago.

I offer this book, *Living Well Naturally,* as a method for nourishing both body and soul, so that you might satisfy in some measure that wholeness which we all seek but which seems to be so elusive.

Anthony J. Sattilaro, M.D.
Philadelphia, Pennsylvania

Part I

Chapter 1

A Change in Lifestyle

YOU ARE FAR MORE in control of your life than you realize. Whether or not you are consciously aware of it, you create your own state of health every day. All you eat, think, feel, and believe dramatically affects your health and happiness. To a great extent, all of us choose to be healthy or ill. We may be unaware of making those choices, but we make them nonetheless. Each day we choose to eat a sixteen-ounce steak, a hot dog, or an ice cream sundae, we make choices about the state of our health. Every day we fail to deal effectively with anger, stress, or depression, we allow ourselves to be driven closer to the precipice we call sickness.

The information in this book will help you make wise choices in your health habits; it will also help you cultivate a positive attitude about yourself, the people around you, and life in general. The program outlined in this book will help you restore your health and prevent serious illness. You will quickly recognize that as your health becomes stronger, you will have more energy and vitality; your thinking will be much more clear and precise; you will feel better about yourself and more capable of handling the challenges that face you; as you become stronger, your attitude about life will be more positive and adventurous. Virtually everyone who follows this

I

program can become more physically attractive. Many will lose weight. If you adhere to the program you should see your blood pressure and cholesterol levels drop to normal, healthy ranges. Your chances of contracting heart disease or cancer will decline precipitously. And this is just the beginning.

I know this program works because my own life was changed by it. In fact, it saved my life.

In June 1978 my physicians told me that I had prostatic cancer, stage IV (D), which had spread to several parts of my body, including my skull, right shoulder, sternum, left sixth rib, and spine. Because I am a doctor, I had access to a great deal of medical information and a lot of free advice. Both the medical literature and the advice drew a pessimistic picture. The scientific studies done on men with prostatic cancer and metastatic lesions divide the odds on survival according to age. Those older than fifty have a good chance of surviving up to five years with the disease. Those under fifty, however, rarely see the five-year mark. For reasons not yet fully understood, prostate cancer in men under fifty is far more lethal; it usually claims the life of the patient within three years after diagnosis. I was twelve days short of my forty-seventh birthday when the disease was discovered in me.

After the diagnosis was confirmed, I underwent three operations during which my left sixth rib and both my testicles were removed. Removal of the testicles — a procedure known as an orchiectomy — eliminates the male hormone, testosterone, which can sometimes slow the spread of the malignancy. In addition, my doctors prescribed regular dosages of the female hormone, estrogen, which can further slow the cancer and sometimes reduce pain.

In my case, the disease was already in its advanced stages. Not only had the tumors spread throughout my body, but I had suffered from acute back pain for nearly two years, a sign that the malignancy could have been with me for some time well before the diagnosis. In light of all of these facts, my physicians advised me that I had between eighteen months and three years to live.

Like many people who have been informed that they have a "terminal" disease, I reacted to the news of my cancer and imminent death with predictable resistance. I denied that I would die; however, the enormous pain I was suffering and the series of operations I underwent quickly made me realize that I was quite mortal and that the worst could happen. Once this harsh realization settled on me, I became depressed — deeply depressed — and resigned myself to a slow agonizing death.

My doctors had hoped that the treatment I was receiving would reduce or even eliminate the pain, but this did not happen. As a result, I began taking narcotic pain relievers, which provided me with several pain-free hours every day, but also caused periodic nausea and vomiting.

While all of this was going on, my father was also dying of cancer. This took an enormous emotional and psychological toll on me. I had to cope with my own disease and with my father's. Perhaps it was most difficult on my mother, who needed a great deal of support but could not always find it in her son.

I seemed to hit absolute bottom on August 7, 1978, the day my father died. His death brought my own mortality into sharper focus; I felt it was a harbinger of my own.

Through a series of providential circumstances shortly after my father's death, I encountered a group of people who were attempting to promote a strange diet and philosophy, which they said would help me reverse my cancer. I was encouraged to begin a diet consisting of 50 percent whole grains (such as brown rice, whole wheat, millet, oats, and barley), 25 percent locally grown cooked vegetables, about 15 percent beans and seaweeds, and the rest made up of soups and various condiments. (The details of how I encountered this diet and philosophy and my recovery from cancer are fully described in

Recalled by Life: The Story of My Recovery from Cancer.) Shortly
after I began the diet, I also took up some simple exercises,
including calisthenics and an Oriental form of yoga exercises
called Do-In. These were very simple and not at all strenuous,
but as I later found out, very effective.

Under normal circumstances I would never have considered following such a foreign and, to my way of thinking,
irrational regimen. Nothing about this dietary and philosophical program made sense to my logical and scientifically trained
mind. This was an Eastern system based on a philosophical
tradition that ran counter to all my medical training. However,
when one is facing one's own death, the beauty of logic and the
false face of pride are among the first things one abandons.
This system offered me a small spark of hope — a priceless
commodity in the face of a death sentence.

One other element in the regimen turned out to be absolutely fundamental to my recovery. The people with whom I
shared this diet and spent much of my time believed implicitly
that I would get well if I followed its precepts to the letter.
There was little, if any, doubt in their minds. Their attitude
provided me with a great deal of support. Ultimately, it was
contagious. Despite my initial misgivings and deep skepticism, I soon began to entertain the thought that perhaps there
was something to this diet and philosophy. Perhaps it could
help me. My skepticism was not easy to deal with, and in fact
has never fully left my consciousness, but I eventually came to
truly hope and have faith in their system. As you will find later
on, belief or faith in recovery is absolutely essential for one to
overcome a serious illness.

About three weeks after I began the dietary regimen, the
back pain I had suffered for more than two years completely
disappeared. I immediately stopped taking the pain relievers.

I could not attribute the pain relief to anything but my new
health practices. Other signs supported this conclusion. For
years I had suffered with digestive problems, particularly
diarrhea. I had been taking a variety of medications for the

problem, including Lomotil, a very powerful pharmaceutical. However, after several weeks of eating my new grain and vegetable diet, my digestive problems also cleared up, and after a couple of months I experienced renewed vitality, along with a deep sense of well-being.

I also lost a considerable amount of weight. After I had begun taking estrogens in June 1978, my weight shot up to a rotund 170 pounds. I used to hover at around 150 pounds, though I preferred to be at about 145. After three months on this diet, I dropped down to 135. Initially, I feared the cancer had returned (weight loss is a sign of advancing cancer), but soon my weight stabilized and I returned to a comfortable 145 pounds. I accomplished this normalization of my weight without having to starve myself, as I had to do in the past. On my new regimen, I generally ate all the food I wanted — within the given limits of the diet.

In addition, I began to take on a more youthful appearance. The deep furrows in my brow and the wrinkles and heavy jowls in my cheeks all disappeared. My face became tight and showed more color. These signs were the antithesis of what a cancer patient normally experiences. I had expected to follow the same pattern that I had seen my father and so many others endure: the endless hours of pain, the enormous suffering, the wasting away, finally bedridden, bloated with drugs, and then, mercifully, death. It is not a death of much dignity.

I was experiencing the exact opposite kinds of symptoms, however. My vitality was improving, my strength was more abundant than it had been in twenty years, my appearance was getting better. At times I simply did not know what to make of it. Could diet, some small exercises, and a commitment to life be enough to reverse this powerful, all-consuming cancer?

By January 1979, blood tests showed that my condition was improving, and by April of that year the tests revealed no sign of cancer. My oncologist, who had followed my progress throughout the ordeal, maintained that my improvement was a result of the orchiectomy and the estrogen treatment.

I could not exclude the possibility that my medical treatment was working synergistically with my own program, but I was beginning to believe that my improvement came about more from my new health habits than from conventional treatment. I was experiencing a rejuvenation far beyond anything one might expect, even with the successful application of conventional treatment.

By June 1979, I felt that I had to prove to myself, as far as possible, what was responsible for my improved condition. I decided to conduct an experiment. Until then, I had been taking estrogens which, in combination with the orchiectomy, was the standard treatment for my cancer. The estrogens had been added to my program at the end of July 1978, about six weeks after my third and final operation. Orchiectomy and estrogens are essentially hormone therapy: one eliminates testosterone, the male hormone, and the other increases the level of the female hormone, estrogen; both are designed to proportionately reduce the level of testosterone in the body, which seems to fan the fires of the cancer. I began the estrogens because the orchiectomy by itself did not seem to be having the desired effect on my cancer; the pain persisted and there did not appear to be a remission.

I felt the only experiment I could safely perform was to stop taking all the estrogens. Any fluctuations in my health might give me some insight into why I seemed to be improving. This experiment could not provide "final" proof that the diet, exercise, and positive attitude were the cause of my recovery, since there was still the orchiectomy, but it would certainly give me more confidence in what I was doing. In the second week of June, I quit using the estrogens; I have never resumed them.

Throughout the rest of the summer I continued to enjoy improved health and well-being. My blood tests that summer showed no sign of cancer, and in August I scheduled a bone scan for September 27, 1979. A bone scan is done by injecting radioactive dye into the blood stream of the patient. In the case of a person with cancer, the dye reacts to tumors by collecting around the cancer and, with the aid of diagnostic equipment, indicates the presence and location of the tumor. In a person without cancer, the dye is spread homogenously throughout the body and is largely eliminated through the urine. It is an extremely accurate diagnostic tool, and has come to be depended on in the recognition of cancer.

My bone scan showed no sign of cancer. There were no aggregated areas of the radioactive dye, and the results of the bone scan — which provides x-ray-like photographs — showed no sign of cancer anywhere in my body. My physicians were stunned. Not only had I arrested the disease, but my bones — which had been filled with cancerous lesions — had completely healed. This is virtually unheard of. As one of my doctors said, bones take a long time to heal. I had been practicing this regimen for twelve months, and it had been only sixteen months since my cancer was detected. This was nothing short of a miracle, I had been told. I was not of a mind to argue.

In the months that followed, I continued to feel strong and healthy; however, I did suffer a couple of setbacks. In April 1980, I contracted a subacute case of thyroiditis and was hospitalized for a few days, during which time a bone scan was performed. (We believed that the cancer had returned and was causing the thyroiditis.) The bone scan revealed no cancer in my body. Through the spring and summer of that year, I continued to feel well, but an October bone scan revealed a small gray spot in my right eighth rib, which I presumed to be cancerous. As it turned out, I was wrong. Another bone scan, on December 27, 1980, showed that the spot had disappeared and there was no evidence at all of the presence of a tumor. Since that time, I have had two more bone scans — one in August 1981, and another in December 1982, both of which demonstrated that there is no sign of the disease anywhere in my body. My blood and liver tests confirm the diagnosis. My physicians have pronounced me to be in a state of permanent remission.

It is now six years since my cancer was diagnosed. According to all the studies and logical conclusions, I should have been dead long ago. Instead, I feel more alive and vital than I've ever felt in my life. I appear younger than I did ten years ago; I have undergone a de-aging process that I did not think existed.

Meanwhile, I have come to love the food I eat; I would not eat any other way, even if I thought my health would not suffer for it. My life is richer and more varied than ever before.

During the last six years I have learned many lessons about health and the wholeness of life. The first, and perhaps most significant, is that we are in a profound sense responsible for our own health. This doesn't mean that we should stop seeing our doctors and begin treating ourselves. Just the opposite. We are responsible for using the information we receive from our physicians and the scientific community to prevent and treat disease.

It is now clear from the abundant scientific evidence that diet is a major cause of the common cancers, heart and artery diseases, obesity, gout, and diabetes. In addition, scientists tell us that these and other illnesses can be prevented through good eating habits.

This year alone, 1 million Americans will die of illnesses of the heart and arteries; another 40 million suffer from such diseases. Cancer will kill more than 400,000 Americans, and another 700,000 people will be diagnosed as having the disease. In addition, millions more will suffer from diabetes, obesity, gout, and other illnesses science terms *degenerative*, meaning that they cause the breakdown of cells or organs. Such diseases have had a crippling effect on our society, causing an enormous loss of creativity, productivity, and money, to say nothing of their impact on our overall happiness.

With simple changes in diet, exercise patterns, and the cultivation of a more positive attitude, these illnesses can be prevented—and in many cases overcome.

Many who are already sick may want to use this program as a complement to traditional therapy, but no one should view it as a replacement for standard Western medical care. My recovery resulted from a multiplicity of factors, including standard medical treatment for cancer, but it is my firm belief that it could not have been accomplished without following the program outlined in this book. But until scientific proof has firmly established that diet and positive imaging can, by themselves, reverse disease, do as I did: use this program to complement your standard treatment.

On the other hand, it's a lot better to stay healthy in the first place, and today we know that correct diet, exercise, and a commitment to life all have enormous and positive effects on health.

My coauthor, Tom Monte, and I have divided the program into three basic and essential parts—diet, exercise, and meditation, or positive imaging. Although each is individually important of itself, no one part could stand alone and have the impact that all three have together. Chapter 8 provides a seven-day program that contains suggestions for meals and times to exercise and use the guided imagery. We recommend that you gradually incorporate these ideas into your life over a twenty-one-day period. We feel confident that at the conclusion of the twenty-one days you'll notice the difference in your health and outlook on life.

We are not talking about health alone, but a recovery of the sense of wholeness, of relatedness to one another and to our common Creator. Once you have established this relationship, there is nothing you cannot do—whether your aim is simply to regain good health or bring peace into your life.

Chapter 2

Your Diet and Health

*I*T'S CLEAR from the scientific evidence that one of the most important factors that led to my cancer was my diet. Growing up, I ate much the same diet that most other Americans consume. If anything, I ate more meat than many Americans because my father was moderately successful in business and could afford such a luxury. As I grew older and became more affluent myself, my diet became even richer. I ate meat three times a day as a rule — bacon or sausage for breakfast, some type of luncheon meat or minute steak for lunch, and roast beef or steak for dinner. I ate fish or poultry only occasionally, and when I did I regarded it as a break from the norm. I enjoyed rich gravies heavy with cream, rolls and butter, eggs, and lots of very sweet desserts. Actually, dessert was my favorite part of the meal, and if my weight was under control I would sometimes treat myself to two. I loved creamy foods in general, and ate a good deal of candy. Doctors eat many of their meals on the run, and chocolate and hard candy are favorites with many physicians. I was no different.

I paid no attention to how highly refined a food was. I didn't

Sources for the information discussed and quotations cited in this chapter are provided in the annotated bibliography.

bother to read labels. I thought one chemical was like another. I put my faith not in my own judgment but in that of others, namely the Food and Drug Administration. It never occurred to me that they might approve foods for general consumption that might not be good for human health. I ate no whole-wheat bread or whole grains, and consumed white bread and refined flour products without a second thought.

I gave no consideration to the fat or cholesterol content of foods. Before I was diagnosed as having cancer, I did not worry much about my heart or my blood cholesterol level. Butter, eggs, meat, dairy products — all of which adversely affect serum cholesterol — were all wonderful, as far as I was concerned — wonderful, that is, until I became conscious of my weight. Then I went back to diligently counting calories, which meant that I ate the same foods, but in lesser quantities.

As for vegetables, I enjoyed mine fresh out of the can or the freezer. As long as my vegetables were tasty — that is, covered with butter or a sauce — I did not complain.

Finally, I ate most of my meals in restaurants. I never really learned to cook, nor had I experienced the joy and creativity that can occur in the kitchen. I considered the kitchen a place for the refrigerator, where I kept some fast food and soda pop on hand. Mine was strictly a utilitarian approach to food and cooking: the faster and more convenient the better.

If this diet sounds remotely similar to your own diet, do not consider yourself abnormal. Unfortunately, you are part of the large majority of Americans whose diets are slowly but inexorably killing them.

The diet most of us eat today is unlike any eaten in the history of humankind. It has sprung up only in the last century and is largely the result of our technology. It is highly processed and rich in fat, particularly animal fat. In fact, studies have shown that between 40 and 45 percent of all our calories come from fat. Foods that are rich in fat include red meat, dairy products, and eggs. The average American consumes about 125 pounds of sugar and drinks 295 12-ounce cans of soda each year. Since many people avoid sugar and soda pop altogether, this means that a vast number of Americans are taking in much more of these two foods than the numbers indicate. The FDA has approved some thirteen hundred different additives for our food supply, not all of which could possibly have been tested for all their short- and long-term side effects. In the past thirty years alone, consumption of artificial colors has increased tenfold. Very few of us eat whole-grain bread and whole-grain dishes. In fact, consumption of whole grains, fresh fruit, and vegetables has been cut in half since the early part of this century. As a result, fiber is virtually absent from our diets.

The grain we do eat comes from white bread and white flour products. These foods have been stripped of their fiber and many of the nutrients during processing, then artificially fortified by reintroducing a few of the nutrients that were removed from the food. However, most of the nutrients that were removed are lost. Meanwhile, much of our food is transported from distant parts of the country or other parts of the world, resulting in loss of freshness and many important vitamins.

Most of us eat a diet that is high in fat, cholesterol, sugar, salt, refined grains, and artificially produced chemicals. On top of this, our food is generally stale. Little wonder, therefore, that salt is suddenly a threat to health; a lot of the taste has simply gone out of our food.

In 1977 the federal government began to fund studies to review the scientific evidence on the role diet plays in the causes of illness. Since that time, three major reports have come out of Washington, D.C., all of which provide a striking indictment against the American diet: *Dietary Goals for the United States* (1977 and 1978); *Healthy People: The Surgeon General's Report on Health Promotion and Disease Prevention* (1980); *Diet, Nutrition, and Cancer* (1982).

These landmark documents say very much the same thing: the American diet is a cause of the leading killer diseases today, particularly the common cancers and cardiovascular disease (illnesses of the heart and arteries, like heart attack, stroke, hypertension, and atherosclerosis).

All three studies urge Americans to change their eating habits and adopt the following general dietary guidelines:

- Eat only sufficient calories to meet the body's needs; in short, do not overeat.
- Eat less saturated fat and cholesterol. These two constituents are found in red meat, dairy products, eggs, the skin of chicken, and some fish. The surgeon general specifically stated that Americans should eat less red meat.
- Eat less sugar.
- Eat less salt.
- Eat more of the complex carbohydrates found in whole grains, vegetables, fruits, beans, and legumes.
- Eat more fish and poultry.

In addition, the National Research Council (NRC) urged Americans to eat more vegetables rich in beta carotene, the vegetable source of vitamin A. Studies have shown that beta carotene may be an effective cancer deterrent, even in people who smoke cigarettes.

Not only should these dietary changes reduce your chances of disease, but other studies indicate that they may improve mental and emotional stability. Recent research done at the Massachusetts Institute of Technology (MIT) suggests that whole grains, particularly, enhance brain chemistry and create a deeper sense of well-being, making one less susceptible to depression and other like emotions.

Let's look at the major elements in our food — fats, cholesterol, protein, carbohydrates, vitamins, and minerals — and their effects on our health. By considering how each of these constituents affects us, we'll be able to understand just what kind of diet will sustain health and contribute to a longer and happier life.

Fats

Fats — an important part of our diet — provide calories, which are converted to energy, and serve in the metabolism of the fat-soluble vitamins, A, D, E, and K. Fats are the most calorie-dense food we eat. A unit of fat has twice the calories of the same unit of carbohydrate or protein, and some foods have far more fat than others.

There are three types of fat: saturated, monounsaturated, and polyunsaturated. Saturated fats are common in such animal foods as red meat, poultry, and some fish and in cooking and baking fats, salad oils, dairy products, and margarine. Unsaturated fats are usually found in vegetables, vegetable oils, and many fish.

Chemically, a saturated fat is different from an unsaturated one in that its string of carbon atoms is saturated, or filled to capacity, with hydrogen atoms. Monounsaturated fats have fewer hydrogen atoms than saturated, and polyunsaturated ones have fewer still.

In general, fat includes two common types — those that are solid at room temperature, like butter, and those that are liquid at room temperature, like oils.

Because fat is so dense, we need only small amounts. In fact, with the sole exception of linoleic acid, a fatty acid found in abundance in oatmeal and vegetable oils, the body can manufacture all the fat it needs from grains, vegetables, and fruits.

Many traditional cultures, such as the Japanese, have subsisted on diets containing as little as 5 to 10 percent of calories in fat, and some cultures have existed on as little as 2 percent. This means that virtually all the fat they eat comes from such sources as brown rice, wheat, barley, other grains, vegetables, and fruit. They eat little or no animal foods and do just fine.

Within the United States, as well, certain population groups — for example, Seventh Day Adventists and vegetarians — consume very low amounts of meat and fat. None of these groups show any signs of illness related to the low level of fat in their diets. On the contrary, the Japanese, the Seventh Day Adventists, and other population groups that consume low-fat diets experience a remarkably low incidence of degenerative diseases, especially heart disease and cancer.

Let's look first at the reasons a high-fat diet causes heart and artery diseases. Studies have shown that dietary fat raises the cholesterol level of our blood. Cholesterol is a waxlike substance used by the body in cell metabolism and as a base for many hormones, and the increase in the cholesterol content of our blood causes the blood to get thick, or sludge.

As the blood becomes thicker and more viscous, it can no longer flow into the smaller veins and capillaries; thus the tissue that would ordinarily be nourished by the flow of blood becomes starved for nutrients and oxygen. Eventually, the tissue dies.

As the blood cholesterol level rises, tiny microns of fat become lodged within the walls of the arteries, particularly those that feed the heart. The particles of fat begin to close off the flow of blood. This disease, in which fat deposits clog the arteries, is called atherosclerosis. As atherosclerosis becomes more advanced, less blood and oxygen make their way to various tissues throughout the body, especially to the heart and brain, causing them to become overworked, tired, and eventually to suffocate. The problem is further complicated by the fact that fat often collects around the heart itself, causing it to work all the harder. Ultimately, the artery (or arteries) is closed off by the fat, and part of the heart or brain dies, bringing on a heart attack or stroke.

A food component that has the same effect as fat on the blood is the dietary cholesterol found in eggs, meat, and dairy foods. Like fat, dietary cholesterol raises the level of cholesterol in your blood and increases the rate of atherosclerosis.

"Only animal foods contain cholesterol in amounts worth talking about," writes nutritionist Patricia Hausman in *Jack Sprat's Legacy: The Science and Politics of Fat and Cholesterol.* "Egg yolk is the most common high-cholesterol food, and organ meats also have large amounts. Shrimp is moderately high. Red meats, poultry, and fish have less cholesterol than these others, but sometimes have much more saturated fat. Both fat and food cholesterol influence blood cholesterol levels, though of the two, saturated fat is more important."

Dairy products, though much higher in saturated fat, also have some cholesterol as well.

Blood cholesterol is measured in milligrams of blood, meaning that a person with a cholesterol level of 250, for example, has 250 milligrams of cholesterol in every 100 milliliters of blood. Such a cholesterol level causes fat deposits to clog the arteries and cut off blood to the tissues. Such persons are headed toward a heart attack or stroke.

Most cardiologists familiar with the evidence suggest that a safe cholesterol level for an adult is under 200. Studies have shown that men whose cholesterol level is 180 or lower have only a small chance of suffering from heart disease. However, as your cholesterol level rises, so too do your chances of heart attack, stroke, and high blood pressure. The chances jump sharply at 250 milligrams and continue upward as the cholesterol level rises. An adult's cholesterol level should not be above 160. This level is relatively easy to attain by simply reducing the amount of meat, eggs, and dairy foods and increasing the amount of whole grains, vegetables, fruit, and small portions of fish or low-fat chicken in the diet.

More than 40 million Americans suffer from the kinds of heart and artery diseases we've just described. Atherosclerosis has been detected in children under the age of ten. Diseases of the heart and arteries kill more than 1 million Americans each year, accounting for one in every two American deaths. These illnesses do more than just kill us, though; they prevent us from working at our best, thinking clearly, and feeling good about ourselves. Never has the world known such a killer disease as this one. Ironically, it is an illness that scientists tell us is almost completely preventable, and even reversible, with proper diet.

Animal studies show that a low-fat diet reduces the rate of atherosclerosis in the coronary arteries — the arteries that feed the heart. No study has examined the effect of a low-fat diet on the plaque (fat deposits) in the coronary arteries of humans. However, scientists have demonstrated regression of artery plaque in humans in the femoral arteries (found in the legs). Other studies have shown that when people consume a low-fat, low-cholesterol diet, their blood cholesterol and blood pressure return to normal range, thus lowering their risk of heart disease and stroke.

You may think that all of this is a sufficient indictment against the standard American diet, but it is only part of the case against the biggest killer loose in our country today.

Recently, the report of the National Research Council, which investigated the link between diet and cancer, stated: "The epidemiological [population studies] and experimental evidence is most suggestive for a causal relationship between fat intake and the occurrence of cancer. Both epidemiological studies and experiments in animals provide convincing evidence that increasing the intake of total fat increases the incidence of cancer at certain sites, particularly the breast and colon, and, conversely, that the risk is lower with lower intakes of fat." The NRC also concluded that fat intake was directly related to cancer of the prostate as well.

Just as with heart disease, countries whose citizens consume high-fat diets have a high rate of cancer while countries whose people eat low-fat diets experience a low rate. In short, research has shown that the more fat in your diet, the greater your chances of getting cancer.

The mechanisms by which fat causes cancer are still unclear. Fat seems to promote the onset of cancer by affecting hormones and carcinogens already present in the body. For example, fat seems to increase the production of the hormone prolactin, which governs milk production and estrogen levels. High levels of prolactin have been found in women with breast cancer, as well as in their daughters, which may provide some clue to why breast cancer runs in families. High-fat diets may cause an aberration in breast tissue and in the endocrine system early in life, thus predisposing women to the disease later on.

In the large intestine, fat seems to cause an increase in the secretion of bile acids and some hormones. Bile acids are secreted by the liver to aid in the digestion of fat; the more fat in the diet, the higher the quantity of bile acids secreted into the bowel. Some scientists say that the bile acids may strengthen the potency of cancer-causing agents already present in the intestines.

Cancer and cardiovascular disease are not the only illnesses associated with a high-fat diet. Fat, of course, causes obesity, a disease that gives rise to a number of other disorders, including diabetes, kidney disease, and gout.

Fat is the most dangerous constituent in our diets today, especially because we eat so much of it. It is clearly wise to cut down on the amount of fat we consume. But how do we do that?

The first place to start is to know which foods are high in fat (see appendix). Most of our fat, by far, comes from two sources: red meats and dairy products. Seventy-five percent of the calories in a lean sirloin steak (with the fat untrimmed) are in fat. Sixty-four percent of the calories in a fairly lean serving of ground beef, or hamburger meat, are in fat. As you can see, as much as three quarters of the calories come from fat. In whole milk 47 percent of the calories are in fat, cheddar cheese 71 percent, and butter 100 percent. More than half the calories in one egg come from fat.

Some fish, like tuna (packed in oil), smoked salmon, sardines, and anchovies, are high in fat, and some shellfish, like lobster and shrimp, are moderately high in cholesterol.

By now you're probably wondering whether *any* foods are low in fat and can therefore be eaten safely. The answer is a resounding yes: all whole grains, such as brown rice, millet, whole wheat, buckwheat, oats, barley, whole corn, and rye; virtually all vegetables and most fruits are low in fat and rich in nutrients. Many kinds of fish also contain safe levels of fat, as does chicken, but only when the fat in the skin has been removed. When I eat chicken I choose the white meat and avoid the skin and the dark meat, which are highest in fat.

It is very easy to avoid a high-fat diet by simply eliminating a few foods, starting with red meat. Because meat is an expensive food, it has become a status symbol in the United States and Western Europe. What is good for status, however, is not necessarily good for health. Most people are unable to eat as much meat as we eat today without suffering from serious diseases. The scientific evidence bears this out time and again.

Many people may not be able to go "cold turkey" and stop eating meat all at once. If you are one of those, do it gradually. Eat small, lean portions of meat twice a week, with the goal of reducing the frequency to once a week. This will help you cut down on your fat intake without forcing you to do something you feel would be impossible at the beginning. Remember that any reduction in the amount of meat you eat will be beneficial, but if you would like to improve your health more rapidly, you should eliminate meat entirely. Do not worry about getting enough protein. You can get all the protein your body needs (see protein section, this chapter) from vegetable sources alone; by eating regular amounts of fish and chicken, you will get additional protein and satisfy your need for animal foods, without the harmful side effects that come with eating meat.

I gave up meat six years ago and have never missed it. For me good health was far more important than enjoying a food I always had trouble digesting anyway.

Try to eliminate all eggs from your diet, since they raise your cholesterol level and increase your chances of illness. Eggs have come to be thought of as America's breakfast food, even though many cardiologists recommend that you don't eat more than two per week. Our program provides delicious substitutes for eggs as a breakfast food and as ingredients in recipes.

Try to reduce and eventually eliminate from your diet milk and all the products derived from it. A large portion of the world's population never eats dairy products. One reason is that many people are lactose intolerant—they have lost the enzyme lactase, which is used by the intestines to metabolize the sugar (lactose) found in milk products. (In many cultures, once children are weaned they eat little or no dairy food during the rest of their lives. People who do not consume dairy products after they are weaned naturally lose the ability to produce lactase, since their bodies no longer need it to metabolize lactose.) Without lactase in their intestines, such people are unable to digest dairy products and suffer from severe digestive problems when they consume those foods.

Cow's milk, of course, is nutritionally inferior to mother's milk for feeding an infant. Cow's milk is designed for the nutritional requirements of a calf, just as mother's milk is designed solely for the needs of a newborn baby. In *Healthy People,* the surgeon general reported:

> Emotional and physical nurturing are vital to an infant's health and breast feeding provides a way of enhancing both ... Human breast milk provides nutritionally complete, convenient, prewarmed food for infants. Breast feeding also increases mother-infant contact, confers some protection from infectious diseases by transferring antibodies from mother to child, and helps women who have gained excessive weight during pregnancy lose it.
>
> Moreover, breast-fed infants rarely are obese and virtually never develop iron deficiency anemia, the most common nutritional problem of American infants.

Of course, aside from being less than optimum sources of nutrition for children, dairy products are high in fat and therefore present all the health risks we've already outlined.

Because many of us were raised on cow's milk, we have come to depend on it as a source of many important minerals and vitamins, particularly calcium, phosphorus, and vitamin D. However, all of these nutrients are available in other sources: green vegetables, seaweed, and sesame seeds are rich in calcium; beans, whole grains, many green vegetables, and whole-grain flour products are rich in phosphorous, and vitamin D is abundant in sunlight, fish, and such fish oils as cod liver oil. (We'll discuss these and other vitamins and minerals later in this chapter.)

For many people, these sources provide adequate amounts of minerals and vitamins. But because of our long-term dependence on dairy foods, and because many people eat haphazardly, some may not be able to avoid dairy foods completely. This is particularly the case with small children, especially those who do not get plenty of sunlight or fish oils. Breast-fed babies have no vitamin D deficiency because mother's milk provides appropriate amounts of all the vital nutrients a baby needs. Once a child is weaned, however, it may need some dairy foods, especially if it shows signs of slow growth or symptoms of rickets. Not all children are able to grow normally without some dairy food or regular amounts of cod liver oil. We should not hesitate to provide these foods to those who need them.

Many adults may feel they need some dairy products, at least during a transition period before they are able to wean themselves completely. But when you eat dairy products, try to do so sparingly, using them as a condiment, and try to confine yourself to such low-fat dairy foods as skim milk and low-fat yogurt. Low-fat yogurt provides many enzymes and natural bacteria that aid in the digestion of food, but these are also provided by the fermented foods suggested in our program.

A great number of people find that dairy products produce mucus in their systems, which gives rise to colds, symptoms of allergy, and sinus trouble. As far as we know, there is as yet no scientific evidence to support this theory. (Some studies do suggest that large quantities of milk cause aberrant behavior in children and adolescents; more research is needed in this area, however). Nevertheless, not everyone has the same reaction to a particular food. Some people handle dairy products much better than others. Our experience with the many people who have used this dietary program leads us to believe that eliminating dairy foods causes a rapid improvement in health. This is especially true in clearing up certain allergies and sinus conditions. But again, this evidence is purely anecdotal, and we suggest that adults experiment cautiously with the consumption of dairy products to discover what, if any, side effects the foods may have on them.

This does not dismiss the important concern one should have over the fat content of dairy food, since fat is clearly the most dangerous constituent in our diets today. *Dietary Goals* and *Diet, Nutrition, and Cancer* both recommended that to reduce the risk of degenerative disease, we should get no more than 30 percent of our total calories from fat. We think this figure is fine for the transition period, but not for a long-term preventive diet. If a number that would represent a safe level of fat intake in the diet has to be assigned, it would fall between 10 and 20 percent of your total calories. This figure is based on the experience of cultures that eat very low levels of fat and show little risk of cancer and heart disease.

Nevertheless, you cannot adequately control the amount of fat in your diet in a piecemeal way, or by expecting a vague percentage figure to provide a clear guide to a safe and healthy diet. The dietary program outlined in Chapter 3 — Your New Healthy Diet — is exceptionally low in fat (between 10 and 15 percent of total calories), and the Transition Diet will help you arrive at this optimum health regimen gradually and at your own speed. The program provides for a substantial reduction of fat in the diet, while ensuring that all the essential nutrients are present in their proper amounts.

Protein

As you look out your window and observe a tree, a blade of grass, or the stem of a single plant, you notice that they all have the strength to stand up straight and the flexibility to bend against the push of the wind. We have the same capacity; protein gives us, and the plant kingdom, this combination of strength and adaptability. Without it, we could not stand up against the resistance of gravity; we would either collapse into an amoebic mass or become so rigid and crystallized that we would shatter into a million little pieces at our first fall.

The protein molecule holds calcium and phosphorous in place; it acts like the skeleton of a building, and the calcium and phosphorous like the bricks and mortar. Protein also forms the basis for our muscles, tendons, and such soft tissue organs as the liver and spleen and aids in the clotting of blood. Protein is everywhere in our bodies — eyes, hair, fingernails, and skin. It accounts for 60 percent of the dry weight of our bodies.

Though protein makes up a very large part of us all, it is not the protein itself that we need in our diets, but the building blocks of protein, called amino acids. Our bodies take proteins from our food — from either animal or vegetable sources — and break them down into their component amino acids. There are literally trillions of proteins, and each of us forms different types, determined by our genetic make-up. Protein is used by the body primarily to replace cells and repair tissue.

There are twenty-two amino acids; fourteen of these are created by the body from a variety of substances, but the other eight can be directly obtained only from particular foods. The latter eight are called the essential amino acids. Many people wonder whether their foods supply complete proteins, that is, all the essential amino acids.

You can get all the protein, including all the essential amino acids, your body needs on a diet made up of whole grains, vegetables, beans, seeds, and fruit. Not all vegetables and grains contain all the essential amino acids, but by eating a variety of grains, seeds, and beans you can be sure to get them all. As long as you eat a whole-grain dish with a common bean, pea, or lentil dish, or with sesame or sunflower seeds, you will get all the essential amino acids and a complete protein. In addition, seeds and beans form a complete protein as well. (We'll discuss condiments and dressings that provide complete proteins in combination with grains or beans in the next chapter.) Vegetarians, who eat no animal food, have no trouble meeting their protein needs. Our diet also includes low-fat fish and poultry, which contain an abundance of protein and all the essential amino acids in a single serving.

Because the purpose of protein is to replace and repair cells, the body needs only small amounts of it. Children need greater quantities of protein for growth and should eat more protein-rich foods.

Many people believe that if they eat lots of protein, they will have lots of energy, but protein makes a very poor fuel because nitrogen is present in the protein molecule. Nitrogen combines with other protein particles to form urea and uric acid, both of which get into the tissues of the body and give rise to gout. Large amounts of protein can be harmful.

Studies have shown that an adult's requirement for protein is between 16 and 20 percent of his or her total calories. When the diet exceeds this amount, the body begins to lose minerals, especially calcium, zinc, iron, and phosphorous, which are leached from the bones and teeth to metabolize the excess protein. The depletion of minerals results in soft teeth and bones and a bone disease called osteoporosis.

In addition, the National Research Council reported that high-protein diets are associated with a greater incidence of cancer, particularly of the breast, prostate, pancreas, colorectum, endometrium, and kidneys.

The average American eats about twice as much protein as the body needs; much of our protein comes from animal sources. Some evidence suggests that protein from animal sources has a much more adverse effect on blood cholesterol levels than do proteins from vegetables.

Now that we know we can get too much protein, is it possible to get too little? In fact, nutritionists have a hard time devising a diet that is adequate in calories to sustain life, yet inadequate in protein. As long as your diet is not made up exclusively of sugar, refined flour, and fat—all of which are filled with empty calories (calories that have no nutritional value)—you are getting enough protein to sustain health.

Our program includes between 10 and 20 percent of total calories in protein, an amount that the body handles efficiently and healthfully. The Transition Diet allows you to eat as much protein as you feel your body needs while you change your eating habits from your current diet to a healthier regimen. Even on the Recommended Diet, however, you can eat high-protein foods, including fish and poultry, and still avoid the harmful effects of fat. You might also try tofu and tempeh, both high-protein soybean foods. (See suggestions in Chapter 3, and the recipes in Chapter 10.) Both foods are highly nutritious, easy to prepare, and delicious.

Try the Transition Diet with the goal of using whole grains, beans, seeds, fish, and poultry as your protein foods. Your good health will be your reward.

Carbohydrates

Like every living and self-propelled thing, the body must have energy to function. Once we become adults, our need for fuel dominates all other dietary necessities. Many thousands of chemical processes take place within the body, and every one of them requires energy. We get this energy from three dietary sources: fat, protein, and carbohydrate. Of the three, the body most prefers carbohydrate: it is the cleanest burning—it leaves behind as by-products only water and carbon dioxide, both of which are easily eliminated by the body. And it is the most efficient source of energy; the body does not have to work very hard to convert carbohydrates into fuel.

Each carbohydrate molecule is called a sugar. Sugars are converted into usable energy by the body and burned as fuel or stored as fat.

The body gets carbohydrates in basically two types of food: starches and sugars. Starches, or complex carbohydrates, are found in unrefined whole grains, vegetables, and fruits. Sugars come from such refined foods as refined grains and simple sugars like common table sugar or sucrose. These two types of foods — complex and refined carbohydrates — have different effects on the body.

Whole grains have been cultivated for the past ten thousand years; they are essentially seeds which, if allowed to, would grow into living plants. Each whole grain is made up of three parts: the germ, which is rich in vitamins, minerals, and some fat; the endosperm, which provides carbohydrate; and the bran, which contains minerals, fiber, vitamins, and protein.

When we eat a whole grain, we get all the nutrients present in the food — not only the carbohydrate for energy, but also the vitamins for metabolism, minerals for healthy blood and cells, protein for cell repair, and fat for the body's energy reserves and vitamin metabolism. The same thing happens when we eat fresh vegetables or fruit, though the proportions of carbohydrate, protein, minerals, vitamins, and fiber are substantially different from those of grain. In other words, we get the entire food and all the nutritional benefits that the body so vitally needs.

With a bowl of brown rice, for example, you are taking in an abundance of complex carbohydrates, or long chains of sugar molecules. These long chains are broken down in the intestines by enzymes, which are produced by the body to stimulate specific chemical reactions such as the breakdown of food for absorption by the intestines. These enzymes begin the process of converting carbohydrates into usable fuel. Each carbohydrate molecule is broken off from the chain, link by link, slowly and deliberately, feeding the body a steady flow of energy. The body is able to control the flow of fuel the way you can control the flow of gas to your car's engine. There are no great shifts of energy — no sudden highs or lows, no 10:00 A.M. or 3:00 P.M. depressions. It is just a steady stream of energy, much like a car traveling at cruising speed on an open highway. It has the effect of providing the body with steady and enduring vitality.

A grain that is refined, however, is stripped of the germ and the bran, and only the carbohydrate is left behind. Food manufacturers often introduce some nutrients artificially and call the food "fortified," but the net effect is a loss of important vitamins, minerals, protein, and fiber.

Refined sugars are in much the same shape. Simple sugar, or sucrose, is artificially extracted from sugar cane and sugar beets, thus separating the sugar from other nutrients that were originally present in the plant.

Sucrose is not broken down in the intestines, as complex carbohydrates are, but is immediately absorbed into the blood stream. When you bite into a candy bar, for example, a great burst of sugar immediately makes its way into your blood stream, causing the overabundance of fuel in the blood stream to be burned and giving you a great rush of energy. However, because the energy is quickly burned, and little or no sugar remains in the blood, you just as quickly feel let down, tired, and sometimes emotionally drained. This condition is called hypoglycemia, or low blood sugar. When it occurs the body is low on fuel and craves energy; people with low blood sugar usually satisfy their craving by eating another candy bar or stick of gum or some other sweet food, which, of course, sets the cycle of highs and lows into motion once again.

Other research has determined that sugar causes a variety of physical and emotional problems. At a Cleveland clinic, Dr. Derrick Lonsdale found that adolescents, who typically eat a diet exceedingly high in sugar and other nonnutritive foods, very often show low thiamine levels and the early signs of beriberi: irritability, mood changes, restlessness, fatigue, depression, insomnia, and chest and abdominal pains. He suggested that sugar appears to be the chief culprit in these symptoms, since thiamine is required by the body to metabolize sugar. As one increases the amount of sugar in the diet, one decreases the body's thiamine levels. When Lonsdale gave his patients more thiamine and instructed them to eat more nutritious foods, their thiamine levels returned to normal and their symptoms disappeared. A study done at the New York Institute of Child Development in 1977 demonstrated that of 265 hyperactive children tested, three-quarters showed abnormal results on a glucose tolerance test. The study suggested that hyperactive children may well have difficulty metabolizing sugar, perhaps exacerbating their condition.

This was the claim made by the late Dr. Benjamin Feingold and the more than fifty thousand parents of the Feingold Association. Feingold maintained that food additives — artificial colors, flavors, and salicylates (aspirinlike substances found in tomatoes, apples, oranges, peaches, grapes, raisins, and some other fruits) — gave rise to hyperactivity in children. Sugar was also implicated as one of the food substances that increased hyperactivity, and recent research indicates support for the Feingold hypothesis.

Dr. Keith Conners of Children's Hospital in Washington, D.C., an expert in the study of hyperactivity, suggests that sugar may well act as a stimulant drug for some children. In an article in the December 1980 issue of *Nutrition Action*, Conners is quoted as saying, "Sugar may act like a stimulant drug in so far as it alters body metabolism. The release of epinephrine that occurs when blood sugar levels rise may have effects similar to those with a stimulant."

Since 1900 Americans have consumed more and more simple sugars as their chief source of energy. Aside from all the conditions we have already mentioned, sugar has been associated with obesity, tooth decay, and diabetes. It also raises blood triglycerides and cholesterol levels, thus contributing to the risk of heart and artery diseases.

Many people feel that eating carbohydrates will cause them to gain weight, but if you get your carbohydrates from whole grains and vegetables you are likely to bring down your weight and keep it there. Simple sugar provides an abundance of empty calories, which tend to be stored by the body as fat. This creates the conditions in which the body puts on weight yet craves nutrition.

Paradoxical as it may seem, many obese people are starving to death. They take in little else but simple sugars and refined grains, which don't supply the nutrients necessary to support bodily functions but do add weight. They are literally starving for vitamins, minerals, and proteins.

Whole grains, vegetables, and fruits are also rich in fiber. Fiber may prevent diseases of the intestines, particularly colon cancer — one of the most common cancers afflicting Americans today. It may also improve intestinal transit time, helping the intestines eliminate toxic constituents that may be working within. It is thought that the longer the bile acids remain in the bowel, the longer they are acted on by intestinal bacteria, which tend to degrade the acids and increase their toxicity.

For centuries doctors believed that constipation was the root of all sorts of illnesses, including cancer. They thought that constipation caused toxins to build up within the intestines and then be drawn into the blood stream, traveling to various parts of the body and creating illnesses at those sites. Although the idea never gained much acceptance, the prestigious British medical journal *Lancet* recently reported that women who suffer from chronic constipation are far more likely to have breast disease, both benign and malignant, than those who have at least one bowel movement per day.

Researchers found that women who had two or fewer bowel movements per week were four times more likely to suffer from breast disease. The scientists also pointed out that the bowels of people who eat meat contain greater amounts of mutagenic substances (agents that cause biological mutation and cancer) than those found in men and women who do not eat meat.

In fact, human intestines are far more like those of herbivores (plant-eating animals) than those of carnivores, or meat eaters. Meat-eating animals have much shorter intestinal tracts, which enable them to digest meat quickly, thus reducing or eliminating the negative side effects that may result from putrefaction in the intestines. The longer digestive tracts of humans, however, may work in exactly the opposite way. Humans may well be ill equipped to eliminate certain types of foods from the digestive tract rapidly, leaving us more vulnerable to foods that putrefy or increase bile acids and mutagenic substances.

By eating fibrous foods, which of course come from plants, we may do a great deal toward preventing serious illness, not only in the intestines, but in other parts of the body as well.

Our program is rich in complex carbohydrates and fiber. Our Recommended Diet is made up mostly of whole grains, vegetables, and fresh fruit. In fact, we recommend that between 70 and 80 percent of your diet be composed of these foods. Our Transition Diet is rich in such foods as well. However you begin Your New Healthy Diet, try to eat at least one whole-grain dish and at least two fresh vegetables a day.

Vitamins and Minerals

A diet of whole grains, vegetables, fruits, and some fish provides an abundance of all the necessary vitamins, minerals, proteins, and carbohydrates for good health. In fact, most nutritionists point out that a vegetarian diet (without any animal foods) made up of whole unrefined foods provides all the vitamins and minerals your body needs, in appropriate quantities, with the possible exception of vitamin B_{12}. Vitamin B_{12} is present in animal foods, including fish and chicken, as well as in tempeh, a fermented soybean product, and spirulina, a seaweed plankton available at most natural food and health food stores.

As long as one eats, it is hard to avoid getting most vitamins and minerals in one's diet. The deficiencies tend to come in a specific group of vitamins and minerals, which we will discuss.

Vitamins

Vitamins are organic substances derived from living tissues of plants and animals. The body uses them to assist enzymes in the metabolism of carbohydrates, proteins, and fats. Like hormones and enzymes, vitamins act as catalysts for chemical reactions within the body. However, the body cannot produce vitamins, as it does hormones, but must rely on the diet to provide them. Because vitamins work with enzymes, they are often referred to as coenzymes. In addition, they often assist in the joining of molecules for the formation of blood and other cells, hormones, and genetic material.

There are more than forty vitamins, but of these only about a dozen are given much attention, since the others are found in abundance and our need for them is small.

The Food and Nutrition Board of the National Academy of Sciences set guidelines for our vitamin and mineral requirements by creating the Recommended Daily Allowances (RDAs). Members of the board point out, however, that the RDAs are only rough guidelines for individual consumption. Vitamin requirements tend to vary with the individual, and the RDAs represent the upper part of the scale, exceeding the required amount for most people. In fact, studies have shown that individual requirements for a particular vitamin can vary by as much as fortyfold.

Certain vitamins, especially vitamins A and D, can be toxic at high levels, and for this reason supplementation can be dangerous. Such fat-soluble vitamins as A, D, E, and K do not have to be replenished every day, since the body is able to store them. Such water-soluble vitamins as B and C do need to be taken daily, however.

We do not recommend that anyone take vitamin or mineral supplements. We view the body as a whole organism whose parts are interdependent; that is, they must work in harmony with one another in order to be fully healthy. Actually, supplementation is a relatively recent occurrence; it has only been in the twentieth century that people began to put vitamins and minerals in pills. The primary source of nutrients throughout history has been the diet, and unless your doctor specifically recommends a vitamin supplement, we suggest that your food be your only source. Supplementation is expensive and usually unnecessary. More important, it can lead to the overconsumption of a particular vitamin, which in many cases can be toxic.

What follows is a rundown of the more important vitamins and minerals, and where you can get them safely.

Vitamin A

Vitamin A prevents night blindness and promotes bone growth and tooth development, healthy skin, hair, and mucous membranes. Recent studies have shown that the vegetable substance used by the body to create vitamin A, called beta carotene, may be an important cancer preventive. The kind of vitamin A found in vegetables is different from the vitamin A (retinol) found in eggs, milk, or liver, which is toxic if taken in high dosages. Beta carotene has not been shown to have toxic side effects, except for a tendency to color the skin orange or yellow if taken in large amounts.

Of all the vitamins in the food supply, none holds out more interest and hope as a possible means of cancer prevention than beta carotene. Remarkably, the studies have found that it seems to protect against cancer even in people who smoke cigarettes, despite the fact that cigarette smoking is the single major cause of lung cancer. This may shed some light on just how powerful a cancer preventive beta carotene may be.

Sources of beta carotene include collard greens, spinach, broccoli, squash, and carrots; cantaloupe, apricots, prunes, peaches, and watermelon.

Vitamin B_1

Known also as thiamine, vitamin B_1 is a necessary constituent in the metabolism of carbohydrates as well as in the normal functioning of the nervous system; deficiencies cause beriberi. Sources of B_1 include brown rice and other whole grains, green vegetables, nuts, berries, peas, soybeans, soybean products, and sunflower seeds.

Vitamin B_2

Riboflavin, or B_2, is necessary for the healthy functioning of cells and metabolism of carbohydrates, proteins, and fats. It also helps maintain mucous membranes. Leafy green vegetables, whole grains, dried beans, peas, sunflower seeds, mushrooms, brown rice, sea vegetables, prunes, and almonds are all rich in riboflavin.

Niacin

Niacin aids in digestion and facilitates energy production by cells. Deficiencies cause pellagra. Sources include whole grains, dried beans, legumes, and nuts.

Vitamin B_6

Pyridoxine, or B_6, aids in the metabolism and absorption of fats and proteins and in the formation of red blood cells. It is also a necessary constituent in the healthy development of the nervous system. Sources of B_6 are green vegetables, whole grains, nuts, potatoes, corn, avocados, legumes, and green peppers.

Vitamin B₁₂

Also known as cobalamine, vitamin B_{12} is necessary to the formation of blood cells and the maintenance of healthy blood and the nervous system. Prolonged absence of B_{12} (it may take years for a deficiency to show itself) causes pernicious anemia, weakness, and lethargy. Sources of B_{12} are all animal foods, including fish and poultry, sea vegetables, tempeh, and other fermented soybean products.

Pantothenic Acid

Also one of the B-complex vitamins, pantothenic acid helps metabolize carbohydrates, proteins, and fats and participates in the formation of hormones. Sources include leafy greens, whole grains, nuts, cabbage, cauliflower, and fruit.

Vitamin C

Vitamin C, also called ascorbic acid, is vital for the formation of collagen — part of the fibrous connective tissue in the body. It may strengthen the immune function, and recent studies indicate that it may well play a role in the prevention of cancer. After reviewing the evidence, the NRC stated that "in general, the data suggest that vitamin C may lower the risk of cancer, particularly of the esophagus and stomach." Leafy green vegetables and citrus fruits are common sources of vitamin C, as are broccoli, sprouted beans, sauerkraut, squash, cabbage, and many tart fruits, such as strawberries. Peppers are also rich in vitamin C.

The NRC urged Americans to eat more fresh vegetables and fruits high in vitamin C.

Vitamin D

Vitamin D is necessary to the formation of healthy bones and teeth, as well as in the body's overall ability to utilize calcium and phosphorous. A deficiency of vitamin D causes rickets; high doses can be toxic, however, and can cause kidney damage, lethargy, and loss of appetite.

The principal source of vitamin D is the sun. The body utilizes sunlight by absorbing the sun's ultraviolet rays and mixing them with cholesterol-like substances just below the surface of the skin; in combination they provide vitamin D. The vitamin travels into the blood stream and ultimately aids in the absorption of calcium and phosphorous through the wall of the intestines.

The most concentrated dietary sources of vitamin D are fish oils, fish liver, and whole fish. Fish obtain vitamin D by eating quantities of plankton, which floats on the surface of the ocean and absorbs sunlight, thereby storing large supplies of the vitamin. Milk and certain milk products, such as butter, are fortified with vitamin D.

The Recommended Daily Allowance for vitamin D is 400 international units, but, as we mentioned earlier, the RDAs were established as general guidelines and were not meant for individual dietary needs. As a rule, infants and children, because they require more calcium and phosphorous for healthy growth, need more vitamin D than do adults.

It is difficult to say how much sunlight is enough to meet the RDA for the average American. In the first place, fair-skinned people tend to process more vitamin D in a given period of time than dark-skinned people, since pigmentation acts as a protective barrier against overexposure to sunlight by shielding the sun's rays. American blacks living in northern cities sometimes suffer from vitamin D deficiency because of a lack of direct sunlight (pollution and tall buildings often obscure the sun, which of course is weaker in the North than in the South during fall and winter months.) As a result, blacks and other dark-skinned Americans may need regular dietary sources of the vitamin.

Authorities typically say that adult Caucasians need only regular or routine sunlight — an hour at lunchtime and a few hours during the weekend — to meet their vitamin D requirements. Since vitamin D is a fat-soluble vitamin, it is stored in the body and does not need daily replenishing.

Infants, of course, also need a dietary source of vitamin D, which is provided in breast milk. Mothers who breast-feed, however, should be sure to get regular amounts of sunlight to ensure that their babies receive adequate amounts of the vitamin. Young children who do not get much exposure to sunlight may also need a dietary source of the vitamin to maintain healthy growth. Should your child show signs of slow growth or rickets, take him or her to your family physician. Your doctor will probably recommend regular amounts of cod liver oil (between a half teaspoon and a full teaspoon provides an abundance of the vitamin) or some low-fat dairy products. You may also want to include regular amounts of fish in your diet and that of your children to ensure the inclusion of adequate amounts of vitamin D.

We should recognize, however, that a high level of vitamin D can be toxic. It can cause kidney stones and demineralization of bones. In other words, be careful with your vitamin D intake at both ends of the spectrum; it is as easy to get too much as to get too little.

Vitamin E

Vitamin E aids in the formation of red blood cells, muscles, and other cells and tissues. Studies have uncovered the possibility that vitamin E plays a role in the prevention of breast disease and cancer caused by nitrosamines (carcinogens found in hot dogs and many barbecued meats). Leafy greens, whole grains, particularly whole wheat, dried beans, safflower oil, and wheat germ are excellent sources of vitamin E.

Vitamin K

Vitamin K is necessary to the clotting of blood and in bone metabolism. Leafy greens, potatoes, cauliflower, peas, soybeans, and soybean products like tempeh and tofu are rich sources of vitamin K.

Minerals

Unlike vitamins, minerals are inorganic substances that come from such nonliving things as rocks. Their roles are similar to those of vitamins, and they are essential to health. Minerals are necessary for cell formation and function.

Again, if you eat a whole-foods diet, you should have no mineral deficiencies. To increase the amounts of minerals and vitamins you eat, it is helpful simply to wash such vegetables as carrots, potatoes, and turnips, rather than peeling them, before cooking. It's also a good idea to cook in a cast-iron skillet, which can help you enrich your foods with iron.

Below is a list of the more important minerals, which are sometimes lacking in highly refined diets.

Calcium

A mineral that is necessary for healthy bones and teeth, as well as for the proper functioning of connective tissue and muscles, calcium can be found in abundance in a variety of green vegetables, which by themselves provide an excellent alternative to cow's milk as calcium-rich food. A cup of milk, for example, contains about 300 milligrams of calcium, while a cup of cooked collard greens has about 320. A cup of cooked mustard greens contains 284 milligrams of calcium, and the same quantity of kale about 206. Green vegetables, as a rule, are all abundant sources of this important mineral.

Sea vegetables are among the richest sources of minerals, trace minerals, and vitamins on earth. An *ounce* of wakame seaweed has about 362 milligrams of calcium. (Seaweeds can be high in sodium; for this reason, they should be rinsed thoroughly or soaked before using. See the section on sodium in this chapter and the information on the use of seaweeds in Chapter 3.)

Finally, sesame seeds provide one of the most abundant

sources of calcium in the food system. One cup of sesame seeds contains 1000 milligrams of calcium. No one is suggesting that you sit down and eat a cup of sesame seeds, but by sprinkling some ground-up, roasted sesame seeds on a bowl of rice one gets plenty of minerals, including calcium, as well as a complete protein.

Phosphorous

Phosphorous is necessary for healthy bones and teeth, as well as muscle formation and function. Good sources are soybeans and soybean products like tofu and tempeh, lentils, beans, chickpeas, sesame and sunflower seeds, whole grains, including wheat and wheat flour, leafy greens, buckwheat, barley, and brown rice.

Magnesium

Necessary for teeth and bones, magnesium can be found in whole wheat, wheat germ, whole grains, leafy greens, soybeans and soybean products, brown rice, lemons, nuts, peaches, and sesame and sunflower seeds.

Iodine

Iodine is essential for healthy functioning of the thyroid gland. Rich sources of iodine include fish, seaweed, Swiss chard, mushrooms, turnip greens, citrus fruits, watercress, and pears.

Iron

Necessary for healthy blood, iron is found in the hemoglobin of red blood cells, which carry oxygen to tissues throughout the body. All animal foods, including fish and poultry, contain iron. Seaweeds are especially rich in iron. Split peas, millet, chickpeas, black beans, pinto beans, prunes, raisins, apricots, wheat germ, and leafy greens are sources of iron as well.

Potassium

Potassium is necessary for healthy functioning of nerves, muscle tissue, and cells. It makes up part of the cells' protoplasm and acts with sodium to conduct electrical impulses through nerve fibers. Potassium and sodium form a delicate balance within the body. When excess sodium is ingested (see sodium section in this chapter), potassium is drawn out from the cells and causes severe fluid retention and swelling, a disease called edema.

Potassium is abundant throughout our food supply, and deficiencies turn up only in people who consume excessive amounts of refined foods or salt. Rich sources of potassium include whole grains, fruit, most vegetables, and animal foods.

Zinc

Zinc is especially important for healthy skin and proper functioning of the sex organs. Seafood, whole-wheat flour, and bulgur are all sources of zinc.

Sodium

For many people, sodium chloride, or table salt, has become something of an addiction, in very much the same way sugar has. In fact, salt and sugar, which dominate the taste of our food, have given rise to a variety of illnesses.

Salt is about 40 percent sodium. The average American eats between 6 and 18 grams of salt per day (about ¾ teaspoon to nearly 2½ teaspoons). Yet our bodies need only about ½ gram of sodium per day, and we can get this and more as a natural component of our food.

Salt has been shown to cause high blood pressure, edema (severe water retention), and cancer of the stomach. Salt seems to have a more pernicious effect on the body when it is coupled with a high-fat diet. Salt and fat apparently combine to increase the chances of illness, particularly cardiovascular disease. High blood pressure, for example, can be reduced simply by reducing the amount of fat in the diet, while keeping salt constant. In countries where diets high in salt are consumed, as in Japan, a much higher incidence of hypertension and stomach cancer occurs.

Dietary Goals, the U.S. Surgeon General, and the National Research Council have all urged Americans to reduce the level of salt in their diets. Foods high in salt include pickles, salt-cured meat, and smoked fish. *Dietary Goals* recommended that we consume only 1 teaspoon of salt per day. At first, this sounds like a reasonable suggestion, but it is nearly impossible to control salt intake if you eat canned and many frozen vegetables as well as meat — even if you never pick up a salt shaker again.

Processed foods are rich in sodium; for many people, these are the primary source of sodium in their diets. Fresh peas, for example, have 0.9 milligrams of sodium; canned peas have as much as 230. These quantities exist before we add salt to our food, or another salted food, butter. Butter contains about 1100 milligrams of sodium per stick (4 ounces or ½ cup). Smoked ham, chipped beef, and smoked fish are veritable sodium mines. One hundred grams of chipped beef, for example, typically contains about 4300 milligrams of sodium, more than 2 teaspoons of sodium or 5 teaspoons of salt.

Eliminate all canned vegetables from the food you eat at home, and eat frozen vegetables only occasionally, to reduce the amount of sodium you take in. (You can get salt-free frozen vegetables, which are richer in nutrition than canned.) We recommend that fresh vegetables be the staples at your table.

Virtually every supermarket in the country has a bountiful supply of fresh vegetables. (See Chapter 3 for a list of vegetables that can be purchased at almost all supermarkets, and should be regulars in your home.) Most fresh vegetables can be steamed in three minutes or boiled in less than twenty. (See Chapter 3 for cooking instructions and Chapter 10 for vegetable recipes.) We also encourage you to vary the vegetables, whole grains, and cooking methods you use to ensure that you get proper nutrition and all the vitamins and minerals your body needs.

A good diet is your best defense against serious illness, but it is more than just protection against disease. If followed closely, our regimen, which is explained in full detail in the next chapter, can increase your vitality, improve your appearance, normalize your weight, and help you sleep more deeply and wake up rested and alert. In short, this diet can make you feel better in body and mind. We do not make this last point lightly.

Increasing evidence indicates that diet can enhance brain chemistry and contribute to improved mental and emotional stability. At MIT, Drs. John Fernstrom and Richard Wurtman have demonstrated that the availability of certain nutrients in the diet can dramatically affect the way the brain works. Writing in *Nutrition Action* (December 1979), a publication of the Center for Science and the Public Interest, Dr. Fernstrom stated, "It is becoming increasingly clear that brain chemistry and function can be influenced by a single meal. That is, in well-nourished individuals consuming normal amounts of food, short-term changes in food composition can rapidly affect brain function."

According to Fernstrom, complex carbohydrates found in whole grains, vegetables, beans, and fruit have the ability to increase the brain's uptake of the amino acid tryptophan, which, studies have shown, aids in the relief of pain and in lowering blood pressure. Tryptophan has also been shown to improve sleep and helps improve mood in emotionally de-pressed people. A diet rich in meat cannot do the same because meat does not increase brain levels of tryptophan.

Shortly after I had begun to follow this diet, I noticed an extraordinary change in my state of mind. Not only had I

experienced all the physical symptoms that have been described here, but I also felt a deepening sense of well-being,
and a growing confidence in myself and my ability to overcome my illness. This was remarkable to me, especially since I
had gone through a prolonged period of despair and depression. I believe the food contributed to my sense of confidence
and well-being. Perhaps the work done at MIT will increase
our understanding of how food affects our minds and emotions, but in the meantime it is wise to use the available
evidence provided us by these and other scientists. The MIT
research is on the frontiers of nutrition science. The work
reported by *Dietary Goals,* the Surgeon General, and the
National Research Council is now well established, and it is up
to us to make good use of such counsel. The next chapter will
explain how to incorporate all this information into a dietary
plan. It will instruct you in ways to gradually introduce certain
foods into your diet while decreasing and eliminating others.
You will find that with a little patience and commitment, you
can easily adopt a new and rewarding way of eating.

Chapter 3

Your New Healthy Diet

C HANGING YOUR DIET is one of the most difficult and challenging things you can do, yet if done right, it can also be one of the most rewarding.

There are two ways to begin a new diet. You could make a dramatic change overnight by replacing all the food in your refrigerator and cupboard today and starting a whole new regimen tomorrow. This doesn't work for most people, and unless you are in poor health and are being counseled by a physician who can help you make wise dietary choices, we do not recommend this approach. You've been building your eating habits your entire life and to suddenly change them one day can be quite a shock, both physically and psychologically. If you don't allow yourself time to adjust to the taste of the new food, or to learn how to prepare it, you may find that you're disappointed by its unusual flavor. You may conclude that you can't go on eating this way and so abandon the entire effort, deciding that the goal was impossible to begin with.

But there is another way: the slow and patient approach, which is far more likely to succeed. By gradually reducing and

Sources for the information discussed in this chapter are provided in the annotated bibliography.

eliminating certain foods while including new ones in your diet, you give yourself the chance to learn how to prepare new dishes tastefully, and the time to adjust to a whole new set of flavors. Meanwhile, there are many immediate and long-term benefits to simply reducing the quantity of meat, eggs, refined grains, sugar, and salt in your diet, and including more whole grains, fresh vegetables, natural desserts and snacks, and an occasional bean or seaweed dish. You only need the willingness to make these positive changes in your life and the patience to let them proceed at a pace that's appropriate for you.

Still, change is never easy, especially in the beginning. Even with death as my shadow, prodding me to make radical changes overnight, I was still confronted with the same cravings and frustrations as anyone attempting to make a fundamental change in diet. When I was first introduced to this new regimen, I was overwhelmed by the enormous changes that were necessary. Because I was very ill, I was instructed to eat a far more restricted diet than the one we are recommending, and I had to start right away. There was to be no transition period. For many months I ate a strict vegetarian diet; I abstained from all animal products, including fish, and ate no fruits or naturally sweetened desserts. (It was not until after my cancer disappeared that I widened my diet to include these foods.) Strangely enough, though I had eaten great quantities of meat throughout my life, I did not miss it in the least when I eliminated it in September 1978. The food I really missed was sugar. For me, dessert had always been the best part of any meal. I was abruptly barred from eating any desserts, including those our own program regards as safe and healthful. Early on, I nearly drove myself crazy trying to satisfy my desire for sugar. I ate huge portions of butternut and acorn squash, both of which are fairly sweet vegetables, particularly when they are baked or pressure-cooked and then whipped into a kind of pudding. I also indulged in great quantities of oatmeal and lentil soup. Despite their delicious flavor—and in the case of squash, the surprising sweetness — these foods will never replace the banana split or strawberry shortcake. Only will power and pure stubbornness saved me. In the end, I decided that survival was more important than satisfying my sweet tooth.

Later, after I began to show some real signs of improvement, I occasionally tried something more daring. I would take barley malt — a malted sweetener made from sprouted barley — and pour it into the bottom of a pot, along with some puffed grain. I'd then heat the entire contents and make a kind of candied puffed grain. After many months of craving a sweet taste, such a food nearly put me in a state of bliss.

That bliss, however, did not last very long. Soon after my initial wave of happiness had crested, I became engulfed by guilt. I immediately feared that this single indulgence had eliminated all the positive steps I had taken. I feared that the cancer was already rising from its embers and about to be set ablaze within me.

This was not the case, however, as my regular blood tests and bone scans revealed. Despite the occasional lapses, my health continued to improve, and I learned two important lessons. The first is that, as much as possible, think healthy. Focus on the improvements and positive efforts you are making, and how they will dramatically improve your health. Recognize these important changes and use them for further improvement. An occasional indulgence will not wipe out all the positive efforts you have made, but the guilt you feel from such an indulgence may well prevent you from continuing on the right track. Guilt serves only to make us feel like failures, and failures have no reason to go on pursuing their goals. Changing your diet is not easy, but if you are to accomplish this goal, you must recognize your progress. Only by feeling good about yourself will you be able to go to the next step.

The second thing I learned is that we should choose less extreme foods to satisfy our cravings. Obviously, some barley malt with puffed whole grain will have a much less severe effect on the body than a banana split. Try to satisfy your sweet tooth with the desserts and snacks outlined below. The same is true for any other craving. Try to eat the food that is lower in fat, cholesterol, sugar, and artificial ingredients. I was surprised to discover how easy it was to satisfy many cravings with healthful substitutes.

Of course, learning to cook these delicious foods will reduce your need to seek nourishment outside the diet. Again, this requires time. You are about to learn to cook foods you probably have never touched, much less put in a pot. Don't expect too much at first. I have never been adept in the kitchen. Cooking an occasional TV dinner or warming a snack was the extent of my culinary experience. The first time I cooked brown rice, beans, and vegetables, I burned the rice, somehow failed to get the beans soft, and turned the vegetables into somethin akin to the swamp weed. It was only through the beneficence of the Almighty that I managed to get beyond these initial failures and stick to the regimen. Needless to say, I have never been sorry.

The joy I feel when I eat this food is still something of a surprise to me, because when I first began the diet I was hostile to it. Unlike many people who change their diets out of conviction or wisdom, I was *forced* to change, or as I thought on other occasions, condemned to it. I was suddenly a prisoner of my food. It took some time before I could get past my self-pity to the point that I could achieve an open mind. Once this occurred, I gradually started to enjoy the food, and after a few months, when my appetite got stronger, I realized that I was actually looking forward to my next bowl of brown rice and steamed vegetables. Even seaweed—which I detested at first—became palatable, and eventually even enjoyable.

The key factors in the program are time and simple willingness. Decide today to create your own healthy diet, and then begin to gradually adopt—at your own comfortable pace—the recommendations we've outlined below.

There are two sets of recommendations. The first is a general series of guidelines that can be used in a transition from your current eating habits to a new, healthier diet. These flexible guidelines are all positive steps and will improve the quality of your diet, and your health. We call this the Transition Diet. Some people may want to stick permanently to this diet, which in itself is a very positive step. The point is that the more natural whole food you eat, the greater your chances of increased health and well-being. How far you go depends on you.

The second set of guidelines is called the Recommended Diet. We consider this the ideal diet, and the one that should serve as your goal. It is not something you must begin tomorrow, or even next month. It may take some people a year or more to get to it; others may decide along the way that this suggested diet does not represent the ideal regimen for them. One should recognize that there is no perfect or standard diet for human beings, but billions of diets, which serve individual needs. We are trying to help you arrive at a diet that is right for you and falls within the nutritional guidelines described in Chapter 2.

Remember, the closer you stick to whole grains, vegetables, beans, sea vegetables, and natural desserts, the more rapidly your health will improve. You should feel an increase in vitality and endurance. You weight should normalize more quickly, as should your blood pressure and cholesterol levels. I believe this diet is one of the best defenses against degenerative diseases such as cancer, cardiovascular disease, diabetes, and others.

We have broken down both programs — the Transition Diet and the Recommended Diet — into nine food categories: whole grains, vegetables, beans, seaweeds (sea vegetables), desserts, snacks, animal foods, beverages, and condiments. The foods listed within each category are highly nutritious and healthful. The only difference between the Transition Diet and the Recommended Diet is that in the former you determine for yourself how quickly you wish to adopt the suggestions, and in what proportions. For example, the Transition Diet allows you to decide how frequently you wish to eat a whole-grain meal per week, while the Recommended Diet instructs you to eat a whole-grain dish at least twice a day. The Recommended Diet makes specific recommendations in all nine food categories.

For both diets, your intake of certain foods should be reduced and, if possible, omitted altogether. Again, the Transition Diet allows you to determine how quickly you wish to reduce or eliminate the following foods.

- All red meat
- Dairy products, especially high-fat foods like whole milk and high-fat cheeses
- Eggs
- Refined flour products like white bread and other refined grains
- Refined sugar like white table sugar and that found in commercially produced foods
- Highly processed foods and foods rich in artificial ingredients

In Chapter 9, we have included a suggested shopping list and a list of kitchen utensils that will be useful in cooking the meals we describe. Chapter 10 contains recipes for preparing the foods listed below.

The Transition Diet
1. Whole Grains

Recommendations
- As often as you can, make a whole grain, instead of a meat dish, the center of your meal.
- Vary your grains among those listed below.

- Whole-grain noodles can occasionally substitute for a whole-grain dish, but cooked whole grain is the preferred food.
- Use whole-grain bread instead of white.

As we pointed out in Chapter 2, a whole grain is unrefined and contains an abundance of nutrients. Refining, however, strips away important nutrients that you would otherwise get from a whole food. Don't be misled into thinking that fortified foods are more nutritious than whole foods just because food companies have reintroduced a few vitamins into the food. Refining results in a net loss of nutrients. A Harvard University agronomist, Professor Paul C. Manglesdorf, says, "A whole-grain cereal, if its food values are not destroyed by the over-refining of modern processing methods, comes closer than any other plant product to providing an adequate diet."

Though we do not recommend that you eat only grains, the point remains that grain is the nearest thing to a complete food. It keeps for years in a cool, dry place and is by far the most versatile of foods. For these and other reasons, whole grains have formed the basis for virtually every civilization in the history of humankind. Manglesdorf writes that "no civilization worthy of the name has ever been founded on any agricultural basis other than [whole-grain] cereals." So dependent are human beings on this singular food that it has become known as the staff of life.

Below is a list of recommended grains and some tips on how to prepare them. See our recipes under Whole Grains in Chapter 10 for more complete directions for cooking a variety of grains.

Brown Rice

Brown rice is perhaps the most ancient of grains. Traditionally cultivated in the Orient, principally in India, China, and Japan, brown rice is now grown throughout the world, including the United States. Rice was brought to the United States during colonial times and was originally cultivated in the South. Today, rice is grown primarily in Arkansas, Louisiana, and California. After wheat, it is the most widely consumed grain in the world.

Brown rice is high in complex carbohydrates, potassium, phosphorous, B vitamins, and niacin. Like all whole grains, brown rice is very low in fat, but contains protein, iron, and other minerals.

Rice can be boiled, pressure-cooked, and fried. To boil, wash the grain thoroughly (it probably has not been washed since it was harvested), place it in a pot of water, add a pinch of salt, and bring to a boil. When the water boils, reduce the heat and allow the rice to simmer at medium heat for about an hour. You may want to add some sliced onions or carrots to the rice while it is boiling.

To pressure-cook brown rice, wash the grain, and for every 1 cup of grain used add 1½ cups of water (for example, 2 cups of rice require 3 cups of water). Add a pinch of salt (no more than a few grains between your fingertips). Fasten the lid on the pressure cooker and place the pot over high heat. The rice will come to pressure in approximately 10 minutes, and the regulator will start to whistle. At this point, reduce the heat to low and allow the rice to cook for 45 minutes; then turn off the heat and allow the pressure to come down naturally. You can speed the process by putting the pot under running water. Remove the lid and put the rice in a serving bowl. Add one of the recommended condiments if you like. (Other grains can be pressure-cooked in the same manner.)

Wheat

Wheat is the most widely consumed grain in the world. It is grown predominantly in the United States, Europe, and the Middle East. Whole wheat is rich in a wide variety of nutrients and contains more protein than rice. Some strains of wheat provide as much as 25 percent of their total calories in protein. Like other grains, wheat is rich in B vitamins and especially rich in vitamin E. It also contains calcium, phosphorous, iron, potassium, and other minerals. Unfortunately, most of the wheat consumed today is refined, and thus is stripped of many important nutrients.

Whole wheat, in the form of bulgur, is extremely easy to prepare and makes a delicious dish. Boil bulgur for 20 to 30 minutes with a variety of vegetables. For every 1 cup of bulgur, add 2 to 2½ cups of water. Cut vegetables (carrots and onions, for example) into small pieces and add them to the boiling water. A few drops of tamari or natural soy sauce can be added to enhance the flavor. Lemon juice or grated ginger root may also be added for flavor. This makes a tasty and nutritious dish.

Barley

Barley is grown throughout the world, especially in Europe and the United States. It is used in stews and can be ground into flour to make bread. Barley is also sprouted to create malt, used in making beer, milk shakes, and a natural sweetener. Barley malt syrup is a rich, sweet syrup used as a substitute for sugar in a wide assortment of dessert recipes. Barley malt can be purchased in most natural food and health food stores.

Barley can be boiled with a variety of vegetables or made into a stew with onions, carrots, celery, and other hearty vegetables. Boiling usually takes about 1 hour. For every 1 cup of barley used, add 3 cups of water and a pinch of salt; boil until the grain is tender.

Buckwheat

Though technically the fruit of a bush, buckwheat has been used as a grain throughout history, particularly in Eastern Europe, where it is used to create Kasha, a hearty and delicious dish. (*Kasha* is also the generic word for buckwheat groats.)

It is boiled with a variety of vegetables, including carrots, onions, cabbage, parsley, and others, for about 30 to 40 minutes. For every 1 cup of buckwheat add about 1½ to 2 cups of water.

The Japanese grind buckwheat into flour to create noodles, or soba. These delicious noodles can be purchased in most natural food stores (see noodle section).

Corn

Whole corn (or maize) has long been a staple grain of North and Central Americans. Highly evolved Indian cultures, including the Aztec, Inca, Mayan, and Hopi societies, were founded on this American grain. When the colonists arrived in America, they used corn to make hasty pudding, hominy, and grits, as well as many other foods. Corn can be ground into flour to make cornmeal for breads and muffins. Cornmeal is also excellent cooked as a grain in a dish called polenta, which is prepared by boiling the cornmeal for about 30 to 45 minutes, shaping the cornmeal into patties, then frying them.

Corn on the cob can be boiled in water for 5 to 8 minutes, or steamed for 10 minutes. Whole corn and corn on the cob, like all yellow vegetables, are high in beta carotene, which, as we have said, may well be effective in preventing cancer.

Millet

Highly nutritious and easily prepared, millet has been used for centuries by traditional peoples of Africa, India, and China. Today it is grown throughout the world, particularly in the United States, where it is used to feed livestock more than it is people. Nevertheless, millet is a highly nutritious grain, rich in carbohydrate, fiber, phosphorous, and potassium. It is also a source of protein, iron, and B vitamins.

Millet can be boiled with a variety of vegetables, especially cauliflower, to create a light and delicious grain dish.

Oats

Oats are a part of European and American tradition. There are several types of oats, including whole oats (the most difficult to prepare because they require the most time), steel-cut oats, and rolled oats. Some rolled oats are more refined than others, particularly those that are commercially produced and packaged. The more refined the rolled oats, the less time they require to prepare, some taking as little as 3 to 5 minutes. The rolled oats that undergo a minimum of processing usually require between 20 and 30 minutes to cook. We recommend that you use the less refined variety, which is richer in nutrition and fiber than the commercially produced and packaged instant oats. Oats are delicious with raisins or currants, or mixed with another grain such as bulgur. The best way to prepare rolled oats is by boiling them; use 1½ to 2 cups of water per 1 cup of oats. You may have to add water if some boils away during cooking.

Rye
Whole rye is used mainly to feed livestock. Most of the rye grown for human consumption is either ground into flour to make rye bread or used as a base for whiskey. Rye bread and whiskey (not necessarily in that order) are, of course, favorites in the Western world.

Noodles
Some whole grains are ground into flour and used to make highly nutritious and delicious noodles. Noodles are a quick and easy way to get grain, since most of them cook in under 20 minutes. We suggest you try to incorporate any of the following whole-grain noodles into your diet. Use them as you would any type of pasta, either plain, with a condiment, in broth, or as spaghetti.

Whole-wheat noodles. A wide variety exists, in many sizes and shapes.

Whole-wheat udon. A Japanese noodle, very much like a spaghetti noodle, with a fine, delicate taste and satisfying texture. Udon is made of a blend of whole wheat and sifted wheat, making it light and easy to digest.

Buckwheat noodles, or soba. Another Japanese noodle, soba is rich and hearty and, like buckwheat, is a highly nutritious food. Soba noodles create their own delicious broth in cooking with a few drops of tamari or soy sauce.

Corn noodles. Light and tasty, corn noodles are made from sifted cornmeal. They are not as heavy as whole-wheat noodles and are wonderful as part of a macaroni dish or salad.

All whole-grain noodles are superior in quality to refined noodles. However, one should read the labels of all packaged foods, including the noodles you buy. They should be made of all-natural ingredients and be free of anything artificial.

Boil noodles as you would any other pasta. Simply add the noodles to a pot of boiling water; add a pinch of salt, some scallions, chives, and/or other vegetables, and boil for 20 minutes or until the noodles are tender.

Use any of the recommended condiments (see the condiment section in this chapter) to season your noodles.

Bread

Few people can resist good bread, and that made of whole grain is by far the most delicious and nutritious bread available. Bread can sometimes contain both salt and oil (fat), two constituents that make it the least preferred source of grain, since salt and oil tend to combine to have an adverse effect on the body. Commercially produced breads made without any salt or oil are available. In addition, once grain is cracked or broken, as in the case of flour, it begins to break down and become less nutritious. Bread will spoil, but whole grain, if stored in a dry place in seed form, can last for years. For this reason, many people choose to buy their own grain mills, grind whole grain into flour, and bake it fresh. This produces the highest-quality breads and is the nearest thing to eating a whole-grain dish.

Please read the labels on bread packaging. Unfortunately, bread has become another product that chemically resembles the package it comes in more than it does the grain that originally went into making it.

A food that can be used in place of bread, but is much lighter, is rice cakes — flat circles of puffed brown rice. They are rich in fiber and carbohydrate and easy to digest. Use them in place of crackers for spreads or jams. Rice cakes can be purchased in most natural food and health food stores and are available in many large supermarkets.

2. Vegetables

Recommendations

■ Vary your vegetables among the three groups — leafy greens, round and ground (squashes and other vegetables that grow near the ground), and roots.
■ Wash, don't peel, such vegetables as carrots, parsnips, potatoes, and radishes. Eat as much of the entire vegetable as possible, for example, carrot tops and turnip greens.
■ Snack on raw vegetables like carrots, celery, cucumbers, and lettuce.

As we said in Chapter 2, vegetables are rich sources of vitamins, minerals, carbohydrate, and fiber. In addition, vegetables are exceptionally low in calories and fat. They are light, delicious, and easy to digest. Because they vary so much in nutritional qualities, we recommend that you vary your vegetables extensively and take full advantage of the variety of the vegetable kingdom.

Of the green vegetables listed below, we suggest that collard greens, kale, mustard greens, and broccoli be used most often because of their rich nutritional qualities. Of the round and ground, all the squashes, cabbage, onions, and Brussels sprouts should be regulars at your table. There are many root vegetables, but of those listed we recommend carrots, turnips, rutabagas, and daikon (a long, white radish originally grown in Japan and now produced throughout the United States). Remember that all yellow vegetables like squash and carrots, and certain green vegetables, like collards and broccoli, are high in vitamin A, or beta carotene, and therefore should be regular parts of your diet.

These and all vegetables can be made tastier by adding quality condiments, like vinegars made from rice and apples, roasted sunflower and sesame seeds, and tofu-based dressings. Grated ginger root also makes a wonderful cooking spice.

Avocados and olives, because they are high in saturated fat, should be avoided.

The nightshade family, especially spinach, tomatoes, peppers, and eggplant, can be acidic vegetables and may cause an adverse reaction in some people. There are numerous anecdotes of people who have found that the nightshade family tends to irritate or inflame arthritis. We know of no scientific evidence for this phenomenon as yet, but those who suffer from arthritis may wish to experiment with the nightshades to see what, if any, effect reducing or eliminating them from the diet has on arthritis pain and inflammation.

Virtually all the vegetables mentioned can be purchased in your local supermarket. They are inexpensive — far cheaper, you will find, than canned or frozen ones — and far more nutritious.

Many natural food and health food stores, farmers' and Oriental markets, carry the more esoteric vegetables. These delicious foods will make your meals more exotic.

Some frozen vegetables on the market are free of salt. Frozen vegetables run a distant second to fresh, but may be used occasionally as a substitute for your fresh foods.

When I first started on this diet, I was bored to tears by vegetables. I soon found, however, that they are special foods — delicious in subtle ways, and highly nutritious. They provide me with a lightness and energy that seem to complement the more filling and chewy qualities of whole grain. The hardest thing I had to learn, however, is that they should not be overcooked.

A list of important and easily obtainable vegetables we recommend you incorporate into your diet follows:

Leafy Greens	*Round and Ground*	*Roots*
Asparagus	Artichokes	Burdock
Beet greens	Bamboo shoots	Carrot
Carrot tops	Beets	Celery
Chinese cabbage	Broccoli	Chicory root
Collard greens	Brussels sprouts	Daikon radish
Curly dock	Cabbage	Dandelion root
Daikon radish	Cauliflower	Icicle radish
greens	Cucumber	Jinenjo potato
Dandelion greens	Green peas	Lotus root
Endive	Leeks	Parsnip
Escarole	Mushrooms	Red radish
Kale	Okra	Rutabaga
Kohlrabi	Onions	Salsify root
Lamb's-quarters	Squashes	Turnip
Leek greens	Acorn squash	
Lettuce	Butternut	
Mustard greens	squash	
Parsley	Hakkaido	
Plantain	pumpkin	
Radish greens	Hubbard	
Scallion tops	squash	
Shepherd's purse	Pumpkin	
Sorrel	Yellow	
Sprouts	squash	
Swiss chard	Zucchini	
Turnip greens	Snow peas	
Watercress	String beans	
	Sweet potatoes	
	Yams	

Methods for Preparing Vegetables

For more specific instructions, see the recipes under Vegetables in Chapter 10.

Leafy Greens

Steaming. Most leafy greens can be steamed in minutes. If you do not have a steamer, simply add ½ inch of water to the bottom of a stainless-steel pot and put in your vegetables. Cover the pot and place it over high heat. Bring the water to a boil, reduce the heat to medium, and steam until the vegetables are done. The length of time can vary, depending on the vegetables and how crisp you like them. Steaming leafy greens usually requires about 3 minutes. (This steaming method can be used for the round and ground and root vegetables as well. The heavier, thicker vegetables, such as Brussels sprouts and carrots, require only slightly more time than the greens, and can occasionally be cooked with greens to form vegetable medleys.)

Boiling. Put water in a pot, add a couple of drops of tamari or soy sauce or a pinch of salt (optional), and bring the water to a boil. Place the vegetables into the boiling water and allow them to cook for 3 to 5 minutes. (You will save a lot of nutrients if you do not place the vegetables into the water until after the water has boiled, since vitamins and minerals are often cooked out of the food and drawn into the water as boiling time increases. Again, you can boil other vegetables in the same way; the cooking time varies with the size and thickness of the vegetable.)

Sautéing. Cut the vegetables into thin strips; brush a skillet lightly with oil (good-quality sesame oil is ideal for sautéing vegetables), add the vegetables, and heat. Sauté for 5 minutes over medium heat; reduce the heat to low and cook for another 10 minutes. You may want to add a few drops of tamari or soy sauce for seasoning.

Round and Ground

Steaming. Steaming is an excellent way to cook Brussels sprouts, broccoli, cabbage, green peas, mushrooms, okra, string beans, and many other round and ground vegetables. Use the steaming method described above for leafy greens. The smaller you cut the vegetables, of course, the faster they will cook.

Boiling. An ideal method for preparing all round and ground vegetables, boiling usually requires anywhere from 3 minutes, for sliced cabbage, to 45 minutes to 1 hour, for sweet squash. Yams and sweet potatoes can be cut into desired sizes and boiled for 30 to 45 minutes. Check the vegetable periodically while it is boiling to determine when it reaches the desired tenderness. Use the boiling method described above for leafy greens.

Baking. Baking is perhaps the best way to prepare all the squashes, yams, and sweet potatoes. To bake squash, first halve the squash, clean out the seeds, and place the open side down on a baking pan or cookie sheet. Bake at 375° to 400°F for 1 to 2 hours or until the squash is tender. Summer squash and zucchini require only about 20 to 35 minutes. Potatoes can be baked by wrapping each one in aluminum foil and placing them in the oven at 375° to 400°F. The amount of time required to bake potatoes varies, depending on the size of the potato; a relatively small potato can require about an hour to bake, while a really large one can require as much as 3 hours. You might also experiment by placing your potatoes in a preheated 450° to 500°F oven and allowing them to bake for 1 hour. This is usually long enough to produce delicious potatoes with crispy skins.

Sautéing. Brussels sprouts, broccoli, onions, green peas, string beans, mushrooms, leeks, okra, and zucchini can all be sautéed with delicious results. Cut the vegetables to the desired sizes and add them to a skillet that has been lightly brushed with oil. Sauté for 5 to 15 minutes or until the vegetables have reached the desired tenderness.

Roots

Steaming. Practically all the root vegetables can be steamed. Use the same steaming method described above for leafy greens; you may add a couple of drops of tamari or soy sauce to the water to enhance the flavor. Root vegetables require more time to be fully cooked — usually between 10 and 20 minutes for radishes, turnips, rutabagas, and some carrots. Probe the vegetables with a fork or taste them periodically to discover when they reach the desired tenderness.

Boiling. Use the boiling method described above for leafy greens to boil all root vegetables. Again, add the vegetables to the water after it has boiled; add a pinch of salt or soy sauce to the water, if desired. Boiling requires anywhere from 10 to 30 minutes, depending on the size and thickness of the vegetable and the desired tenderness.

Baking. Baking is an ideal way to cook root vegetables. Cut the vegetables into the desired sizes and place them in a casserole or baking pan that has been lightly coated with oil; if you would like to omit the oil, add about 1 inch of water to the bottom of the pan, along with a stalk of kombu seaweed, if desired (the seaweed adds minerals and flavor to the food).

Sautéing. Slice root vegetables into the desired sizes and sauté them as you would other vegetables. Sautéed root vegetables are wonderful when they are mixed with such vegetables from the other two categories as onions, mushrooms, Brussels sprouts, and collard greens.

Broiling. Carrots, turnips, potatoes, and rutabagas are ideal for Vegetable Shish Kebab. Place the vegetables on a skewer and broil them in the oven or over a barbecue grill, basting occasionally with a mixture of water, sesame oil, lemon juice, and, if desired, some tamari or shoyu (natural soy sauce) to enhance the flavor and keep them from drying out. Other ideal foods for Vegetable Shish Kebab include tempeh, a soybean patty we'll describe later, tofu, also a soybean product, and seitan, or wheat meat (see recipes under Whole Grains in Chapter 10). Fish and chicken can also be broiled with vegetables.

3. Beans

Recommendations

- Cook beans with a stalk of kombu seaweed (see the Seaweed section in this chapter) until they are very tender to improve their digestibility.
- Use tofu, tempeh, and other bean-based foods as regular substitutes for bean dishes. Both tofu and tempeh can be cooked within 15 minutes, and tofu can be eaten raw.

Beans are the greatest single vegetable source of protein. When eaten with a whole grain or sunflower or sesame seeds, beans provide us with a complete protein, which is to say that we get an abundance of all the essential amino acids. Beans also supply high amounts of vitamins, minerals, carbohydrate, and fiber. Not only are they rich in nutrition, but they are also delicious and satisfying foods.

Only whole grain has provided humankind with a more versatile food source. It would be impossible to list all the foods beans are used to create. Among them are felafel, a Middle Eastern dish made with chickpeas, and hummus, a creamy delicious spread for sandwiches and crackers, also made from chickpeas but bearing no resemblance to its distant cousin, felafel. Tofu, tempeh, soy sauce (or shoyu) tamari, and miso are all made from soybeans, and all bear a uniquely rich taste and high nutritional value.

Tofu, a soybean cake, is rich in protein; it can be purchased in many supermarkets, as well as natural food and health food stores. Tofu may be eaten raw or cooked and used as a base for a wide assortment of foods, from dressings to desserts.

Tempeh, a soybean product that comes in six-inch-square patties, has a cheeselike flavor and consistency; it is rich in protein, as well as vitamin B_{12}. Tempeh can be steamed, boiled, broiled, and fried in minutes; it can be used in stews and soups and is wonderful with noodles. Tempeh is a fermented food, and thus is rich in digestive enzymes. It is carried by most natural food and many health food stores.

The U.S. Department of Agriculture's *Composition of Foods, Agriculture Handbook No. 8* compares the nutrient content of tofu and tempeh with ground beef. The figures are striking. Tempeh has more protein than ground beef (19.5 percent protein to 17.9 for ground beef), nearly twice the iron (5.0 milligrams for tempeh, and 2.7 for ground beef), and nearly a third as much fat (7.5 grams per 100-gram serving for tempeh; 21.2 grams of fat per 100 grams for ground beef). Tempeh compares favorably in practically every other category as well. It has more phosphorous, vitamins A, B_1, B_2, B_{12}, and niacin than ground beef. Ground beef has 70 milligrams of cholesterol per 100-gram serving, while tempeh has none at all. This is true of tofu too; it is a nutritionally rich food, but is low in fat. When one realizes that both tempeh and tofu are easy to prepare and convenient, one begins to appreciate the real value of this delicious food.

There are literally hundreds of different types of beans; several nutritious kinds are listed below. We have also provided some general advice for cooking beans. Be sure to see the recipes under Beans in Chapter 10 for more specific instructions on how to prepare individual dishes.

Azuki

Originally the prize of the Orient, especially Japan, azuki beans are now grown in the United States, most notably in Ohio. The small red azuki bean is rich in protein, carbohydrate, and B vitamins. It also contains iron and vitamin A. The beans can be boiled and pressure-cooked with a stalk of kombu seaweed in the pot. They can be cooked together with brown rice for a delicious and nutritious dish. Grains and beans, of course, provide a complete protein, so all the essential amino acids are present.

Black-eyed Peas

Black-eyed peas are regarded as a delicacy in the southern United States, where they have long been part of the good southern cooking tradition. Black-eyed peas are rich in protein, carbohydrate, and B vitamins.

Black Soybeans

Originally grown in the Orient, black soybeans eventually migrated westward, where they remain a popular food to this day. Delicious and rich in nutrition, black soybeans are easier to digest than their cousin, the yellow soybean.

Chickpeas

Also called garbanzo beans, chickpeas are a staple food in Italy, Spain, Central America, and the Middle East. Chickpeas are the basis for such popular Middle Eastern dishes as felafel and hummus. The large golden beans are delicious boiled by themselves or with sliced carrots and onions added. Chickpeas are rich in protein, carbohydrate, B vitamins, and iron.

Kidney Beans
Large red beans shaped like a kidney (hence their name), kidney beans have long been a favorite in Mexico and in the southwest United States. Kidney beans may be eaten alone or used as a base for soup.

Lima Beans
Very popular in Mediterranean countries and eaten widely across the United States, lima beans make delicious soups and stews. Besides being rich in protein and carbohydrate, lima beans provide an excellent source of vitamin A and calcium.

Lentils
Popular throughout the Middle East, lentil beans are reputed to be depicted in ancient Egyptian wall hangings that date back to twelve hundred years before Christ. Lentils are part of the traditional Jewish cuisine, as well as a popular food with many Americans. Lentils are among the easiest and fastest beans to prepare; you can boil them in 45 minutes to 1 hour and have a delicious, high-protein food. Lentils are among the easiest beans to digest; they make an excellent introduction to this food if you are not used to eating beans. Lentils are a good vegetable source of iron.

Navy Beans
The beans that became famous for being baked, navy beans are regarded as an all-American food. Unfortunately, they are often served with frankfurters. Navy beans, as all beans, are delicious with whole-grain bread and make wonderful stews. They are a rich source of protein, carbohydrate, and calcium. Navy beans also contain iron and B vitamins.

Pinto Beans
A traditional bean of the southwest United States, especially Texas, the small white pinto bean is delicious cooked alone or

in combination with carrots and onions. Pinto beans have protein, carbohydrate, and, along with lentils and chickpeas, are a good source of iron.

Soybeans

One of the most revered foods of the Orient, soybeans have been used to make an incredible array of foods. Tofu, tempeh, natto (a fermented bean dish with a rich, exotic flavor), and miso (a soybean paste used as a base for soups and dressings, which is rich in digestive enzymes and nutrition) are just a few of the foods made from soybeans. Soybeans by themselves are difficult to cook, since they require so much time, and hard to digest. Most of the soybeans grown in the United States are used to feed livestock. Yet traditional peoples in the East recognized the wealth of nutrition in soybeans and used them as a base for naturally processed foods. Tofu and tempeh are becoming increasingly popular in the United States as people search for high-protein foods that are low in fat and cholesterol. Miso, a fermented soybean product like tempeh, is used as a base for various types of vegetable soups, but can be moderate to high in sodium. However, low-sodium misos that are rich in digestive enzymes and nutrition are available. If you decide to use miso, we recommend that you choose a low-sodium variety and use only ⅛ to ¼ teaspoon of the paste per bowl of soup, to ensure that you get smaller amounts of sodium while enjoying the abundance of vitamins and minerals available in miso. (See the Bean section of Chapter 10 for a recipe for Miso Soup.)

Split Peas

Among the easiest beans to cook and digest, split peas are delicious as a basis for soups and stews. Cook them with carrots and other root vegetables, onions, and some wakame seaweed (optional) for a hearty and delicious soup/stew. Split peas contain protein, carbohydrate, and iron. They are also high in beta carotene, the vegetable source of vitamin A.

Methods for Preparing Beans

Boiling. Boiling is the preferred method for cooking many beans. Soak the beans overnight and boil them with a single stalk of kombu seaweed, if desired. Add a pinch of salt (a few grains between your fingers will be enough) or a few drops of tamari or shoyu when they are 80 percent done. (Taste a few beans to see if they are nearly done.) Most beans take about 1 ½ to 2 hours to cook. (Beans keep well in the refrigerator, so they can be cooked the night before and refrigerated until dinnertime or kept for several days during the week. They can then be taken out of the refrigerator and reheated in minutes.)

Pressure-cooking. (Before you pressure-cook beans, be sure the regulator escape valve is clean and that no obstructions are present to prevent the pressure from escaping from the pot.) Wash the beans, put them in a pot with kombu seaweed, add 3 cups of water for every 1 cup of beans, and cover the pot. Place over high heat until the beans come to pressure (usually within 10 minutes). Reduce the heat to low and cook for 45 minutes. (The regulator should issue a low hissing sound throughout the cooking period, indicating that the beans are being cooked under pressure. This ensures that the nutrition is being locked into the food.) When the time is up, wait for the pressure to come down or put the pot under cold water to bring down the pressure quickly. Remove the cover, season the beans with a few drops of tamari or shoyu, and boil for about 30 minutes or until the beans are done.

Baking. Place the beans in a pot of water; for every 1 cup of beans, add 3 to 4 cups of water, and boil with a stalk of kombu seaweed, if desired, for 15 to 20 minutes to loosen the skins of the beans. After this is done, pour the beans and the water into a baking pan or bean crock, cover, and bake at 350°F for 3 to 4 hours. When the beans are about 80 percent done, you may add a variety of condiments or spices, such as raisins or miso soybean paste, to make the flavor richer. Add water to the beans during the baking period whenever necessary. Keep the beans moist — they should be soft and creamy when finished.

In a rush? Tofu and tempeh can be cooked in a variety of ways — from steaming to boiling — within 10 to 15 minutes. Tofu is precooked and can be eaten raw with sliced scallions, grated ginger root, and a drop of tamari on top.

Beans are rich and satisfying foods. Among the beans listed, azuki, lentils, chickpeas, split peas, and pinto beans are highly recommended for their nutritional qualities and robust flavor.

4. Seaweeds (Sea Vegetables)

Recommendations

- Try incorporating seaweed as a side dish; use only small amounts of seaweed — up to 1 tablespoon per serving.
- Try seaweeds in soups and stews instead of using them as a side dish. This will help you get used to their initially foreign flavor.
- Rinse and/or soak seaweeds thoroughly before using them, to remove as much of the sodium as possible.
- People who take medication for hypertension should eat only small portions of seaweed (1 teaspoon) once a week and eliminate all meat, dairy products, eggs, and canned vegetables from their diet. They should also refrain from using all condiments that contain sodium.

For centuries, humankind has been harvesting the sea, drawing from its depths an incredible array of rich and exotic vegetables. Seaweeds are harvested from coastal waters all over the world. The Maine coast produces alaria, dulse, kombu, wild nori, kelp, and others. In Japan, where sea vegetables have been farmed for centuries, seaweed production has been turned into a high art. The Japanese produce arame, hijiki, kombu, wakame, agar (a natural gelatin excellent for dessert recipes), and many others. The Irish produce Irish moss and dulse, and the French Corsican moss. Seaweeds are farmed in New Brunswick, Canada, and in Africa.

Futurists and visionaries have always looked to the sea as a major source of food for a growing worldwide population. And with good reason. Seaweeds are among the most nutritious foods known to humankind. One hundred grams of hijiki seaweed (less than 4 ounces) contain 1400 milligrams of calcium, 56 of phosphorous, and 29 of iron, and 150 international units of vitamin A. Seaweeds are also rich in iodine, magnesium, zinc, and many trace elements. One does not have to eat great quantities of seaweed to derive these enormous benefits. On the contrary, one should eat only small portions of this high-potency food because it is high in sodium. For this reason we urge you to rinse and soak seaweed before you use it. Used wisely and in moderation, sea vegetables can be a great boon to your diet and to your health.

If you live near coastal waters, you can harvest your own seaweeds. The best place to collect them is in rocky waters, especially in places where a rocky shoreline continues into the water. Seaweeds can be collected in the shallow pools formed by rocks and jetties. If you are new to seaweed harvesting, you'll want to start by harvesting only those seaweeds that grow in the calm waters, near the shore; however, seaweeds are best collected in the more active waters, which tend to produce cleaner sea vegetables. Generally speaking, two people are required to collect seaweeds—one to go into the water, cut the seaweeds from the rocks and ocean floor, and the other to put them in bags or baskets while keeping an eye on the tide. Seaweeding is done at low tide, which exposes the sea vegetables sufficiently to be cut. While doing this, however, one tends to forget about the tide, which can be dangerous because the waters can suddenly become deep or the currents change. Several excellent books—among them *The Seavegetable Book* by Judith Cooper Madlener; *Seaweeds* by C. J. Hillson; and *Seaweeds at Ebb-Tide* by Muriel Lewin Guberlet—provide information on how to gather seaweeds, their traditional uses, nutritional content, and how to prepare them tastily.

Below is a list of sea vegetables we encourage you to incorporate into your diet. See our recipes under Seaweeds in Chapter 10 for detailed instructions on how to prepare them. *The Seavegetable Book* provides not only an excellent introduction to seaweeds and seaweed harvesting, but also many fine recipes. Remember to soak seaweeds for at least 30 minutes before preparing them.

Alaria (Alaria esculenta)

Found in North Atlantic coastal waters, alaria, also called edible kelp, is related to the Japanese wakame. It can be cut into small pieces and steamed for 30 minutes with carrots, onion, daikon radish, and other hearty vegetables. It can also be used in soups and stews. Alaria is high in B vitamins, vitamins C and K, carbohydrate, and many trace elements.

Arame (Eisenia bicyclis)

Arame, a delicious Japanese seaweed that can be used as a vegetable (steam with carrots, onions, and lemon juice) or in soups and stews, is stringy and tender and can be cooked in 20 to 30 minutes. It is rich in protein, carbohydrate, and vitamins A and B; it also contains many minerals, including calcium, iron, sodium, potassium, and trace elements.

Dulse (Palmaria palmata)

Dulse is found in temperate waters on both the Atlantic and Pacific coasts. It can be eaten in many ways: raw, marinated in lemon juice, steamed with other vegetables, or in soups and stews. Dulse, which is a leafy seaweed, can also be roasted and ground for use as a condiment, or lightly steamed and eaten as part of a salad. Dulse is high in protein, vitamins A, C, E, and B vitamins. It also contains fat, iodine, and a variety of minerals and trace elements.

Hijiki (Hizikia fusiforme)

Hijiki, a rich, stringy seaweed shaped like noodles and grown off the coast of both Japan and China, can be boiled with a variety of vegetables for 1 to 1½ hours. Carrots, onions, and daikon radish are excellent complements to hijiki, which is high in protein and contains carbohydrate, fat, vitamin A, B vitamins, calcium, phosphorous, iron, and many trace elements.

Irish Moss (Chondrus crispus)

A sea vegetable harvested off the Atlantic coast for centuries, Irish moss has traditionally been used as a natural thickening agent in soups and stews. It is a constituent in traditional Irish cough medicine. High in vitamin A and iodine, Irish moss also contains protein, carbohydrate, vitamin B_1, iron, sodium, phosphorous, calcium, and many other minerals and trace elements.

Kombu

Kombu appears in several varieties, the most common of which comes from Japan (*Laminaria japonica*). It is used in cooking beans (to help soften the beans; many people find it makes them easier to digest) and, as a vegetable, cooked with onions, carrots, rutabagas, turnips, and daikon. Kombu comes in stalks and is easy to use in a wide variety of ways. It is one of the most nutritionally rich sea vegetables, high in protein, potassium, vitamin A, B vitamins, iron, sodium, carbohydrate, fat, and many trace elements.

Laver (Porphyra perforata)

Found from the Polar Regions to the South Temperate Zone of the Pacific Ocean, laver (also known as summer seaweed and sea lettuce) has been used traditionally by American Indians and the Japanese. Laver can be sautéed or used in soups and stews. It is high in the B vitamins, vitamin C, protein, and carbohydrate.

Nori (Porphyra tenera)

Nori grows off the coasts of both Japan and the United States. In the Orient, nori is harvested and flattened into sheets, which are dried and used to wrap rice to form sushi (rice rolled in roasted nori seaweed) or rice balls (balls of rice wrapped in roasted nori). The nori harvested from the North Atlantic and east coast of the United States, also called wild nori, grows into leaves and may be eaten alone as a vegetable or in soups and stews. Wild nori can be sautéed with carrots, onions, and other vegetables in 15 to 20 minutes, and both the wild and Japanese varieties can be roasted in minutes and ground to provide a delicious condiment for whole grains. Nori is one of the most nutritious of seaweeds. It is very high in vitamin A, protein, carbohydrate, and B vitamins. It contains vitamins C and D, calcium, phosphorous, iron, and many trace minerals.

Wakame (Undaria pinnatifida)

A rich, tender sea vegetable, wonderful in soups and stews, wakame is a leafy seaweed that also can be cooked by itself or with other vegetables. Simply soak the wakame for 20 minutes, cut it into small pieces, and boil (add just enough water to cover) with vegetables of your choice. Add lemon juice and sesame seeds as condiments.

These sea vegetables are available in most natural food and health food stores. They are easy to prepare and, as we have shown, nutritional gold mines. In addition to the sea vegetables described above, there is a seaweed product called agar, or agar-agar, which is used as a thickening agent in desserts and sauces. Tasteless and colorless, agar is the ideal natural gelatin. It too can be purchased in natural food and health food stores.

5. Animal Foods

Recommendations

- When you desire animal foods, eat fish as your first choice and chicken as your second.
- Eat fish that are low in fat.
- Remove the skin and fat before and after you cook chicken.
- Eat the white meat of chicken; it is much lower in fat than the dark.
- Occasionally use fish or chicken in soup for a light and easily digestible way to eat these foods.
- When you dine out, request that your fish be cooked in as little butter and salt as possible.
- Avoid fish that is high in fat, such as swordfish, whitefish, bluefish, mackerel, and salmon.

See the recipes under Animal Foods in Chapter 10 for ways to prepare fish and chicken. The following fish are low in fat and cholesterol: sole, halibut, haddock, flounder, cod, snapper, tuna packed in water, and brook trout.

Most shellfish contain low to moderate amounts of fat, but some, like lobster and shrimp, are high in cholesterol. Scallops are low in fat, but are often prepared in a great deal of butter. However, if you adhere closely to the program, an occasional small portion of seafood is not apt to be a problem.

6. Condiments and Dressings

Recommendations

- Use the condiments listed below on whole grains, vegetables, and salads.
- Avoid all highly processed condiments, as well as salt (except very small amounts in cooking) and pepper.

We suggest the following condiments and dressings. (See the recipes under Condiments and Dressings in Chapter 10 for more specific instructions.)

- Sesame seeds, roasted and ground into a fine powder. Sprinkle on whole grains as you would table salt.
- Sesame seeds and small fish. Roast and grind sesame seeds in combination with any of a number of small dried fish, such as dried sardines or chirimen iriko; the sesame seeds and fish can be ground in a number of ways: with mortar and pestle, in a suribachi—a bowl with a rough, serrated interior—with a pestle, or in a blender. The fish can be ground separately, then added to the sesame powder. This condiment should consist of approximately 10 parts sesame seeds to 1 part fish. This high-protein condiment provides vitamin D and many other vitamins and minerals.
- Sesame seeds and seaweed. Roast and grind sesame seeds in combination with ground roasted kombu, dulse, or nori. This condiment should consist of approximately 10 parts sesame seeds to 1 part seaweed.
- Grated ginger root. Excellent on tofu, soups, and stews. Ginger root can be purchased in virtually any supermarket, as well as most natural food and health food stores.
- High quality rice or cider vinegar
- Roasted sunflower seeds. Excellent on vegetables and grain.
- Tofu-based salad dressing (see page 203).
- Orange or grapefruit slices. Wonderful on fish or chicken, as well as on bean dishes. Orange juice or grapefruit juice can be mixed with miso to form a delicious salad dressing. Use only a small amount of miso with warm orange juice and pour over salad.
- Oil and vinegar
- Lemon juice, or sliced lemon, as on fish
- Fish flakes, like bonito, in soups and stews
- Horseradish
- Scallions, chives, and parsley
- Natural shoyu and tamari. Shoyu, or natural soy sauce, and tamari are traditional condiments of Japan. They are made from soybeans, which are cooked and then allowed to age naturally, without the use of chemicals to speed up fermen-

tation. There are distinct differences in taste and processing between the two condiments; shoyu is made directly from soybeans, while tamari is a by-product of miso, another fermented soybean product, which includes grain in its recipe. Both shoyu and tamari contain sodium — between 17 and 18 percent of their total composition. This is less than half that of table salt. Though natural shoyu and tamari are less harmful than salt, they should nonetheless be used with discretion. We do not recommend that you add either of these condiments to your food at the table; however, both are excellent in cooking. A few drops are all that's necessary to amplify and enhance the natural flavors of your food.

Traditionally made shoyu and tamari contain no artificial ingredients. They are naturally aged and brewed with care by master craftsmen in Japan. Both products are rich in digestive enzymes and bacteria, and the Japanese have long held that small amounts of shoyu and tamari (don't use them together) aid digestion.

We urge everyone who would like to use these products to purchase them from reputable natural food producers. Many of the soy sauces on the market today — especially those found in typical Oriental restaurants — are mass produced and contain a wide range of highly suspect additives and chemicals that are used to speed up aging and provide flavor.

7. Snacks

Recommendations

- When you snack, use unrefined, natural foods.
- Avoid snacks that are cooked with excessive amounts of oil, salt, and sugar or have been stripped of their fiber and subjected to artificial ingredients, as are most of the heavily processed snacks on the market.

Since snacking is done on impulse, it is a good idea to keep healthful snacks available in your home. Natural foods will at least provide unadulterated sustenance when you feel the urge to eat "something." A list of suggestions for healthful snacking follows.

- Dried fruit
- Raw vegetables, such as carrots, cucumber, celery, and others
- Rice cakes
- Popcorn (without salt or butter)
- Puffed grain
- Natural candies made without sugar, such as yinnies, which can be purchased in most natural food and health food stores, along with many other kinds of natural snacks and desserts
- Good-quality whole-grain bread
- Sunflower, pumpkin, and sesame seeds (try roasted seeds combined with raisins and other dried fruit)
- Natural, unsweetened apple butter and other fruit spreads with rice cakes or whole-grain bread.

8. Fruits and Desserts

Recommendations
- Substitute natural, whole-food desserts (made from whole grain and natural sweeteners) for sugary, commercially produced desserts.
- Use fruit, fruit juices, barley malt, and yinnie (rice) syrup instead of refined white sugar as sweeteners for cooking.

Dessert is clearly one of the most enjoyable and satisfying parts of any meal. We recommend that the sugar you eat be a natural constituent of your food, as in the case of fruit, or that a mild natural sugar, such as those listed above, be used with a whole-grain dessert (for example, Oatmeal Cookies made with oatmeal, raisins, and sweetened with apple juice or barley malt; carrot cake made with whole-wheat flour, carrots, and sweetened with any of the natural sweeteners).

We recommend that you choose natural desserts, which do not cause such extreme reactions in the body as huge bursts of insulin from the pancreas, and provide needed nutrition as well as carbohydrate or sugar.

The desserts we recommend, and others you can create along our guidelines, will provide you with satisfying flavor and rich nutrition. For starters, see the recipes under Fruits and Desserts in Chapter 10 for cooking instructions. A list of suggested dessert dishes follows.

- Fresh fruit.
- Cooked fruit, like baked apples or pears.
- Fruit crisp. Sliced fruit cooked with rolled oats, raisins, sunflower seeds, and any one of a number of available natural sweeteners (fruit juice, barley malt, or yinnie syrup).
- Homemade applesauce. Peeled and cored apples (and/or other fruit) boiled until tender and puréed. Cinnamon, nutmeg, and other mild spices may be added.
- Kanten. A gelatin dessert made with fruit, fruit juice, and agar seaweed. (See recipe under Fruits and Desserts in Chapter 10.)
- Oatmeal and other whole-grain cookies. Oatmeal, with a little whole-wheat pastry flour, raisins, and barley malt or apple juice as a sweetener.
- Couscous Cake. A cake made from partially refined wheat. (See recipe under Fruits and Desserts in Chapter 10.)
- Fruit pies. Apples, cherries, strawberries, blueberries, or any other fruit can be used to create delicious pies, using whole-wheat flour instead of white, fresh fruit instead of sugared and canned, natural sweeteners instead of sugar. The same can be done with most cake recipes.

There is no limit to the number of delicious and healthful desserts you can create with a little imagination.

9. Beverages

Recommendations

- For optimum health, refrain from drinking beverages that contain caffeine, sugar, and artificial additives.
- Avoid iced or excessively cold drinks; they shock the system and tend to upset digestion.
- If you drink alcohol, do so in moderation, and try to drink only high-quality natural beers and wines that have been brewed or fermented naturally and contain no sugar or artificial ingredients.

We suggest the following drinks for regular consumption:

- Roasted grain coffee substitute made of roasted barley and other grains.
- Spring water
- Kukicha (bancha) twig tea, which can be purchased in most natural food and many health food stores
- Vegetable juices
- Fruit juices

This is the Transition Program, which gives you a set of general guidelines for healthy eating. Chapter 8 provides a recommended meal plan for seven days, and Chapter 9 includes a shopping list of foods that produce healthful meals. Use these foods to replace your standard fare to the extent that you feel comfortable with them. Make the Recommended Diet Program, which follows, your goal. This will encourage you to make regular changes in a safe and healthful direction. Remember to go at your own pace, and refuse to allow an occasional setback to keep you from achieving your goal: a safe and health-promoting diet.

The Recommended Diet is the best regimen we can offer. It is one which we believe most people can and will follow eventually, given the time and a deeper understanding of nutrition and healthful cooking. The Recommended Diet is composed of the same nine food groups as the Transition

Diet, except that here one attempts to restrict one's eating only to those foods outlined below. For brevity's sake, we will occasionally direct your attention to specific foods discussed earlier in the Transition Diet rather than repeat the same information.

The Recommended Diet

1. *Whole grains.* Eat a whole-grain dish at least twice a day. Whole grains, including whole-grain noodles and breads, should make up between 40 and 50 percent of your diet.
2. *Fresh vegetables.* Eat at least four cooked vegetable dishes a day. Vegetables should make up 25 to 30 percent of your diet.
3. *Beans.* Eat a bean dish three to four times a week; beans should make up about 10 percent of your diet.
4. *Seaweeds.* Sea vegetables may be eaten two or three times a week as a side dish or in soups and stews. Eat only small amounts of seaweed, approximately 1 tablespoon per serving, except that those who are on medication for hypertension should limit the amount to 1 teaspoon once or twice a week.
5. *Animal foods.* We recommend that if you eat animal foods, you choose fish first and chicken second. Limit fish to once or twice a week and chicken to once or twice a month.
6. *Condiments and dressings.* Use ground roasted sesame seeds and the many recommended condiments (see the list of condiments under the Transition Diet). Do not use table salt, pepper, or commercially produced condiments and dressings.
7. *Snacks.* Raw vegetables, rice cakes, salad, small portions of seeds with dried fruit, and other healthful snacks may be eaten daily in moderation (see the list of snacks under the Transition Diet).

8. *Fruits and desserts.* Cooked and raw fruit or whole-grain desserts with a fruit or natural sweetener may be eaten once or twice a day.
9. *Beverages.* Drink beverages that contain no caffeine, sugar, or artificial ingredients. (See the list of recommended beverages under the Transition Diet.)

At first, the Recommended Diet may appear excessively restrictive, but we assure you that you can learn to enjoy the food on this diet just as much as you do that of your current one, except that our diet will keep you healthier. All you have to do is become familiar with the tastes of the food and the various methods for preparing it. If you make a serious effort to follow the Transition Diet, you will automatically find yourself developing a taste for whole grains, vegetables, beans, sea vegetables, and natural desserts. Eventually, these foods will become so familiar to you that you will find they make up the greater portion of your diet. In short, you will be well on your way to following the Recommended Diet, and doing it painlessly.

Consult the shopping list in Chapter 9 for help in obtaining the foods you need to begin the program. Most of the foods on the list can be purchased in your local supermarket, and all of them can be obtained in natural food stores. If you have never shopped in a natural food store you will probably find this list useful.

So far we have said a lot about food from a scientific perspective, which has provided the basis for this sound and healthful diet. But there is much more to eating — indeed, to living — than our rational, scientific approach would indicate. Before the twentieth century and the ascendency of modern science, people lived and chose their foods according to a more subtle, if inexplicable, faculty we call intuition. Survival was based on humanity's ability to live in harmony with the land and the greater cycles of the earth — the weather patterns and the seasons. Although traditional peoples suffered from various infectious diseases and illnesses arising from poor sanitation, their rates of degenerative diseases were low to nonexistent. Thus, there is something good to be said about our ability to make instinctual dietary choices. Today, science has replaced the traditional wisdom of the past, yet we continue to make some of our food choices on the basis of our physical relationship to the environment. We prefer light foods, such as salads, fruits, and cool drinks, in the summer and hot, heavier foods, such as soups, stews, and breads, in the winter. Most of us eat differently in the morning than we do at night, and if we are wise we abstain from eating for a few hours before going to sleep each night. We regard these intuitive responses as common sense; we do not need a double-blind study to tell us that they make a difference in our comfort and health.

Let your own intuition and common sense be your guide in incorporating into your life the information provided in this book. Because food is so intimately connected to our physical comfort each day, it soon becomes the basis for our sickness or our health, our prison or our freedom. Don't let our dietary program become a conceptual prison for you; use the information we have provided as guidelines for better eating to put you on the road to improved health. Give careful consideration to what we have said, chew it well, digest it, and make it your own. By following the guidelines slowly and thoughtfully, you will come to know beyond any doubt which foods make you feel well and which leave you feeling poorly. Over time, you will learn to manipulate the diet to meet your more subtle needs as well, for example, whether you prefer more vegetables, less grain, or more fish on a given day or week than the program outlines. If you work with this program, your body will soon tell you what it needs. Don't think that variety, the very spice of life, will forsake you the minute you embark on this diet. You will find that even in the Recommended Diet there is incredible flexibility in the kinds of dishes you can prepare and the frequency with which you can eat certain foods.

Finally, food isn't everything, not even in health. Our environment, our behavior, and our faith in ourselves and the larger forces of the universe all play important roles in our health and happiness. Food has an important place in this larger picture, and it can do a great deal to increase our health and bring more harmony into our lives.

Chapter 4

Your New Exercise Program

SHORTLY AFTER I began the dietary program outlined, I also started an exercise routine. Although I had little faith in what I was doing at the time, I nonetheless accepted the idea that my only hope of surviving rested with my adopting the program completely. The exercises included walking, calisthenics, and a series of Oriental exercises called Do-In, which are based on the principles of acupuncture. These three types of exercise, I found, were very effective in creating fitness, relieving tension, and increasing vitality.

Isotonic or aerobic exercises, which improve the heart, circulation, and lung capacity, are best for most people. These types of exercise include walking, jogging, bicycling, swimming, and calisthenics that stretch muscles and increase the intake of oxygen (knee bends, toe-touching, jumping jacks). Isometric exercises, such as weightlifting, push-ups, and other exercises that set muscles against heavy or immovable objects, do not improve the conditioning of the heart and can even be dangerous to those with heart disease. Aerobic exercises cause us to breathe deeply, providing more oxygen to the lungs,

Sources for the information discussed and quotations cited in this chapter are provided in the annotated bibliography.

heart, and the entire body. When the heart is exercised, it pumps more blood per beat; that is, it works more efficiently and is gradually strengthened through regular exercise. One of the clear signs that your heart is becoming stronger is that your pulse begins to slow down. This means that the fibers that surround the heart and cause contraction and expansion are becoming more coordinated. They are able to expand together, allowing more blood to flow into the heart's chambers, and contract together, pumping more blood out of the heart with a single beat. As the beats become fewer per minute, the heart is allowed more time to rest. The difference between 90 beats per minute and 60 is that at 60 the heart is able to rest twice as long between beats.

The average adult man's heartbeat rate is around 72 per minute, while the average woman's is about 76. Generally speaking, anyone whose heart beats more than 80 times per minute when the body is at rest is in poor health, and is headed for a heart attack.

Exercise not only brings down the number of heartbeats per minute; it lowers blood pressure as well. Exercise tends to eliminate the stickiness of blood platelets — the small colorless disks that travel through the blood and aid in clotting. When one consumes a high-fat diet, these platelets become sticky and begin to sludge, or thicken, preventing them from flowing smoothly through the smaller veins and capillaries. As noted in Chapter 2, this prevents the blood from nourishing various tissues that depend on these tiny capillaries to supply blood. Without blood the tissues die. Reducing or eliminating the stickiness of the platelets is an important step toward better circulation. (Exercise will not lower blood cholesterol levels, however, and cholesterol levels are most responsible for the sludging of the blood and the onset of atherosclerosis. Your new diet will lower your blood cholesterol level and, coupled with exercise, will dramatically improve circulation.)

Exercise that involves the legs is particularly important. As the muscles in the calves relax and contract with exercise, they act as auxiliary pumps. During relaxation, the muscles absorb blood; as they contract, they push blood back to the heart. This type of continuous action takes a great burden off the heart. Walking is an excellent example of an exercise that strengthens the heart at the same time it improves circulation by working the leg muscles.

Exercise also improves blood circulation to the brain and helps dissolve blood clots throughout the body, including the lungs, heart, and brain.

All exercise, of course, burns calories and eliminates fat from the body. Active people look trimmer because their muscles are tighter and more compact. Compared to muscle, the same volume of fat appears loose and saggy.

Of course muscles that are not used begin to atrophy or disintegrate. Interestingly, the same is true of bones; without exercise, we tend to lose calcium, and our bones become weak and brittle and more vulnerable to fracture. Studies have shown that exercise is great for relieving tension and helping control compulsive appetites. A brisk half-hour walk will do more for the health of your heart, your peace of mind, and your out-of-control appetite than any pill yet invented. However, the reverse is also true: the data show that less exercise is associated with increased tension and greater appetite.

People who exercise regularly and vigorously talk about a natural "high" they experience. But even moderate amounts of exercise will provide you with deep relaxation and better sleep. You will also experience a greater feeling of confidence and a sense of well-being.

According to exercise experts, you need only ten minutes of exercise three days a week in order to be well on your way to excellent physical condition. In fact, the best gauge for the effectiveness of your exercise is your own pulse. Those who are in sufficiently good health should perform exercises that raise their pulse rate to 120 beats per minute for at least two minutes at a time; in addition, one should exercise for at least thirty minutes per exercise session. This is not a particularly strenuous pace for a healthy adult; the maximum number of times the heart can beat per minute is approximately 220. At that point, the heart doesn't work any more rapidly regardless of the level of stress it's under.

Nevertheless, it is important for anyone who plans to start an exercise program to see his or her physician before beginning. This is especially important for those who suffer from any type of chronic illness, such as cardiovascular disease, diabetes, and arthritis.

Walking

Perhaps the best exercise of all, and clearly one of the safest, is walking. Experts tell us that half an hour of brisk walking is enough to condition the entire system, especially if your pace is between three and five miles an hour. Not everyone can get up to that speed right away, so let yourself approach it gradually.

You should try to get in at least one brisk half-hour walk per day. Immediately on setting out, you will feel your heartbeat pick up. You will breathe deeper and exercise your entire cardiovascular system, lungs, and much of your muscular system. If you feel you cannot sustain a brisk pace, try to maintain a higher speed for at least two minutes and then slow down to a more comfortable pace for a while. After a short rest, pick up speed again and maintain it for two more minutes. Do ten of these quick two-minute intervals, or simply maintain the same brisk pace for a twenty-minute period or more. Either of these methods will provide you with an excellent conditioning exercise.

Walking is one of the best exercises for relieving tension and restoring equanimity to the mind. Tension can be thought of as excess energy that's trapped. Certain organs begin to race — the heart beats faster and the stomach secretes excess acid; blood pressure rises. When you walk, you put your whole body in motion, thus quickly and efficiently burning excess energy. Your systems calm down; heartbeat and blood pressure return to normal. Tension dissipates. All aerobic exercise, including walking, is excellent for relieving stress and its negative side effects. (We'll talk more about stress and how to deal with it in the next chapter.)

Walking is therapeutic in ways that you cannot anticipate, particularly if you can walk in calm surroundings, like a park or a country setting. Even in a city, amid the teeming profusion of so much energy, you can gain a certain anonymity, fade into the crowd, and let your tensions be carried off by the great rush of life that hurries down Main Street.

Of course, walking also burns calories. A mile of walking burns as many calories as a mile of running. The difference is that running a mile better stimulates the cardiovascular system, lungs, and muscles, since it places more stress on them. Still, for those who have not exercised for some time, or do not enjoy jogging, walking is by far the next best thing.

Actually, we were built to walk—we are perfectly structured for it—and there is no reason, short of handicap, why most of us cannot take advantage of this wonderful and health-restoring exercise. It costs nothing and requires no partner (although it can be a very sociable activity as well). It provides great benefit and enjoyment, and it's free for the taking.

In addition to walking, I also do calisthenics three or four days per week. These are short stretching exercises, briefly described below, that take no more than ten or fifteen minutes in the morning or evening.

Calisthenics

Knee Bends

Turn the back of a chair toward you, and hold the chair for balance. Keep your back straight, breathe in, and bend at the knee until your buttocks rest against your heels. Now, stand up straight and, as you do, exhale, completing the round. Remember to breathe deeply throughout this and all exercises. Do this ten times or as many as you feel comfortable doing. Do not strain yourself. Try to maintain the exercise for at least two minutes.

Bending at the Waist

With your hands on your hips, bend at your waist, bringing your torso down toward your knees; bend as far forward as you can without straining. Keep your hands on your hips while doing the exercise (do not reach for your toes). You should feel a mild stretching of the hamstring muscles in the backs of your legs, calves, and Achilles tendon. Now, come back to an upright position and lean backward as far as you can, stretching the muscles in your chest, stomach, and thighs. Come back to a standing position, completing one round. Do not strain yourself. Do this five to ten times, maintaining the exercise for at least two minutes.

Leg Lifts

Lie down on the floor. Bend your knees and bring your feet to your buttocks, so that your feet are resting flat on the floor with your heels as close to your buttocks as possible. Remain with your back to the floor. This is not a sit-up. Now, extend your legs straight out again, hold them up for a moment, as they are pointing straight out, and rest them on the floor, completing one round. Do this ten times or as many as you feel comfortable doing. Do not strain.

Side to Side

Stand up, with your legs shoulder-distance apart. Bend as far as you can to your immediate left, then as far as possible to your immediate right. Come back to an upright position. One round includes bending once in each direction. This stretches the abdominal muscles, particularly the sides, where we often have excess fat, or what is commonly called love handles. It also stretches the back, chest, and shoulders. Do this ten times, or as many as you feel comfortable doing. Remember to breathe deeply throughout the exercise, and maintain a consistent pace for at least two minutes before resting. Do not strain yourself.

These exercises are designed to increase oxygen intake and exercise the heart and muscular system. They are not strenuous, but they are effective.

Three seasons out of the year, I ride my bicycle regularly. Bicycling is an excellent aerobic and cardiovascular exercise, to say nothing of the workout your legs get.

Remember that all movement is in a sense exercise. All one is attempting to do with walking and calisthenics is intensify the experience over a shorter period of time. Half an hour a day of walking (more if you can do it) and ten minutes a day of calisthenics for three or four days a week will provide you with an abundance of exercise and dramatically reflect itself in your health.

Once you begin to exercise regularly, you'll find yourself naturally getting more exercise without giving it much thought. This is one of the reasons you should start out slowly. If you strain yourself, exercise quickly becomes painful and unrewarding. However, if you are patient and gradually work your way up to a more demanding pace, you'll be more likely to stick with an exercise program. Meanwhile, you'll be getting stronger and better able to increase your pace without straining yourself. Before you know it, you'll be parking your car a distance from your destination just so you can walk, or taking the stairs rather than the elevator, recognizing that you have a hundred wonderful opportunities each day to get short but intensive workouts.

The third type of exercise I perform is Do-In, an exercise/massage based on the principles of acupuncture. Do-In is often referred to as *acupressure* massage, because it uses finger pressure and exercise in place of the acupuncturist's needles.

It is helpful to understand acupuncture in order to appreciate Do-In.

Acupuncture has been practiced in China and Japan for more than two thousand years and endures to this day as one of the most common medical practices in the East. Using only small, thin needles, which are inserted into the skin just below the surface, acupuncturists claim they can effectively treat virtually any illness. Acupuncture has been proved to be an extremely effective pain reliever and anesthetic, though few people in the West understand why it works. As for its efficacy as a treatment for illnesses, little is proven.

The World Health Organization states that acupuncture is an effective treatment for as many as forty illnesses, and acupuncturists themselves claim to be able to treat diseases of the nervous system, gastrointestinal tract, blindness, deafness, arthritis, and severe headaches, among others.

Acupuncture has only recently gained recognition in the Western world, and particularly in the United States. Actually, acupuncture did not come to the West until the sixteenth century, when missionary doctors brought back the practice from Asia to Europe. Acupuncture began to catch on in the United States during the last ten or fifteen years. Its growing popularity is due in a large measure to the reporting of *New York Times* columnist James Reston, who experienced its effectiveness firsthand. In 1971, when he was traveling in China, Reston suffered an appendicitis attack and had to be operated on in Peking. The operation proved successful; however, following the surgery Reston began to suffer from "considerable discomfort, if not pain." A Chinese acupuncturist was sent to minister to him. The acupuncturist inserted three needles into his right elbow and one below each knee. He also burned some herbs over Reston's stomach, while "manipulating [the needles] in order to stimulate the intestines and relieve the pressure and distention of the stomach," Reston later reported. He said he experienced a "noticeable relaxation of the pressure and distention within an hour and no recurrence of the problem thereafter."

Following his recovery, Reston toured a number of Chinese hospitals, where he witnessed the use of acupuncture as an anesthetic in several major operations, one of which was performed on a man for the removal of a brain tumor. During the operation, the patient was "perfectly conscious"; he talked with Reston through an interpreter and ate orange slices while his "skull was laid open." In another remarkable example, Reston observed an operation on a man who had a "vast gaping hole" in his back, through which he could see "the gasping" of the patient's lung. What astonished the reporter all the more was the fact that only one acupuncture needle was used to bring about anesthesia — in the patient's right shoulder. Again, this man was perfectly conscious and conversed with Reston during the operation.

Reston was understandably impressed by the effectiveness of the acupuncturists and their small needles. He wrote, "There is enough objective evidence of practical medical information in the use of acupuncture to justify exploration ..." He concluded that "something is really going on here, and it is clearly too important to be left to newspaper reporters."

Following Reston's report, many American medical doctors visited China and substantiated Reston's observations on the validity of acupuncture as an anesthetic. Critics of acupuncture, meanwhile, have tried to argue that it is mere hypnosis. However, this view has suffered repeated setbacks from studies showing acupuncture's effectiveness under controlled conditions. Nevertheless, many medical authorities remain unconvinced, and others call for more studies to confirm the clinical observation.

Several theories try to explain how acupuncture may work. Some scientists suggest that it may stimulate the autonomic nervous system, thus affecting pain and various types of illness. Others maintain that the needles cause the body to secrete endorphins, a morphinelike substance created by the body, which gives rise to pain relief and mild euphoria. (We'll talk more about endorphins in the next chapter).

Neither of these explanations addresses the questions of why the needles must be inserted at precise locations and how these locations, or points, have an effect on distant parts of the body (for example, three needles in Reston's elbow and a couple below his knees caused pain relief in his stomach).

Only the traditional view of acupuncture attempts to explain these questions, but as yet it is not getting much attention since there is no theoretical basis or experimental evidence for it in Western medicine. That theory says that human beings live within a field of energy, which surrounds and permeates the body and flows along certain distinct pathways called meridians.

Practitioners of traditional Oriental medicine believe that twelve meridians run vertically throughout the body, like twelve deep rivers. Points that correspond to organs and organ systems are located along each meridian. The acupuncturist inserts a needle into one of these points, using it like an antenna to direct energy into a specific organ via the point and meridian that he or she has chosen.

An Oriental healer sees health as a state in which energy flows freely along these meridians; that is, there is no blockage or stagnation along the energy pathways. Blockage of energy results in a symptom — either pain or an illness. The blockage acts like a dam, causing energy to increase in one place and decrease in another. The needles are used to modulate the imbalance, directing energy to the weakness and draining it from the area where it is excessive. This is done by the placement and manipulation of the needles. Early Oriental philosophers developed the practices of yoga and Do-In from this theory of energy.

Do-In uses massage techniques and stretching exercises to attempt to eliminate blockages along these energy pathways. Instead of using needles at various points, one massages the points, or attempts to stretch the meridian itself to stimulate energy flow along the meridian and unblock the stagnation that may be causing the problem.

This is a controversial area, of course, and although there is some small support for acupuncture in the West simply because it seems to work, there is no evidence of which we are aware for the efficacy of Do-In. Although I have no rational explanation for it, I can report that my personal experience with Do-In has been rewarding, and I encourage you to try the Do-In exercises and hope you may benefit from them as well. The exercises are safe and easy. They place little or no stress on the body, and anyone can do them. All the Do-In massages should be performed gently and thoughtfully. Try to focus on what you are doing—that is, try to "see" a particular organ or organs relaxing or becoming more vital. This will also help stimulate improved health, as you will learn later, when we discuss the impact of the mind on the body. Let's review the exercises, and see if you don't feel increased health and vitality through doing them regularly.

The Do-In Exercises

Sit in a comfortable chair that will help keep your back straight. Breathe deeply and try to relax. Rub your hands together vigorously for a couple of minutes. They should soon feel warm. Circulation should increase and you should feel a kind of low vibration in them. Now, follow the steps outlined below.

Your Head

Lightly tap your entire scalp with your fingers or very loosely clenched fists for about 2 minutes. It should be a gentle, even pleasant sensation. When you are through, rub your face vigorously, concentrating on your forehead, cheeks, nose, and chin, for another 2 minutes.

The head and face are considered to be places where many acupuncture meridians are found. By stimulating these points, acupuncture theorists say, one sends energy to many organs in the body. I always feel a bit more clear-headed and mentally keener once I've done this exercise.

Your Shoulders

Again with a loosely clenched fist or the fleshy part of your hand at the base of your thumb, gently but firmly pound on your shoulders, from the base of your neck out to the edge of your shoulder for about 2 minutes. Use your right hand for your left shoulder and your left hand for your right shoulder. Lightly pound each shoulder for about 2 minutes.

According to acupuncture theory, the large intestine and lung meridians run along the top of the shoulder. By pounding on these meridians, acupuncturists maintain, one increases energy and vitality to these organs.

Your Arms

When you have finished pounding your shoulders, come down to your arms, either vigorously rubbing or pounding them, again with a loosely clenched fist, for about 2 minutes. You should massage your arms so that you come down toward your hands along the outside of each arm, and come back toward your chest along the inside of each arm. By doing this, it is said, one helps the natural flow of energy along the meridian. Do several repetitions on both arms.

The meridians located in the arms are the heart, lungs, small intestine, large intestine, and two general meridians that are associated with the functioning of the cardiovascular system.

Your Hands

Again, rub your hands together vigorously for about 1 minute and then shake them, as you would a mop, for another minute.

(Readers with arthritis may just want to rub the backs of the hands and palms, and forgo the rest of the exercise.) With your right hand, take your left thumb, rotate it clockwise for a few revolutions, then pull on it slightly and let it go. Do the same for each finger on both hands. Again with a loosely clenched fist, pound the palms of both hands, especially the center of your palms, for about 1 or 2 minutes. This is said to stimulate energy to the heart.

A number of important meridians and acupuncture points are located in the hands; they include the heart and circulatory system, the large and small intestines, and lungs.

Your Chest

With loosely clenched fists, lightly pound the upper part of your chest for about 1 minute. This should be done gently, and there should be no pain. If you find this or any exercise painful, discontinue it immediately.

Massaging the chest is believed to stimulate the heart and lungs.

Your Legs

Pound the outsides of your legs with a loosely clenched fist, going downward along the outside of each leg, from your hip to your foot, and then back up the inside of each leg, from your foot to the top of your thigh for about 1 minute. Take another minute to massage your thighs and calves thoroughly with your thumbs.

It is believed that the meridians located in the legs include the bladder, kidney, stomach, gall bladder, liver, and spleen. Again, by pounding or massaging these meridians, one is said to be stimulating energy to these specific organs.

Your Feet

Rub your feet vigorously for 1 or 2 minutes, then pound the bottoms of your feet for several minutes. This will increase the circulation in your feet and tends to relieve fatigue.

The feet are another area of major importance in acupuncture because so many important meridians are believed to be located here. Among them are the liver, spleen, stomach, gall bladder, sex organs, and kidneys. By massaging the feet, one is presumably stimulating and vitalizing these organs. Tired feet, according to Oriental medicine, indicate general body fatigue, and a good foot massage can do much to relieve tension and mental and physical fatigue.

The entire exercise routine should take you no more than 10 to 15 minutes. It can be done at any time of day, and almost any place. Remember that the exercises should be done gently and thoughtfully. You may feel a dull ache associated with the massage, such as you would get from a good shoulder massage. If you feel more than that amount of pain, discontinue the exercise. I believe that by doing the exercises regularly and thoroughly, you will soon see an improvement in your health and vitality.

There is absolutely no scientific explanation for the benefits to be derived from these exercises, but at worst they are harmless and at best they may work for you as well as they did for me and the thousands of people in the East who have practiced them since ancient times. So try them anyway, as part of the program described in Chapter 8. You should have no trouble fitting them into your schedule, and you may be surprised by their effectiveness. Couple these with a daily brisk walk and Your New Healthy Diet, and you will be well on your way to a rebirth of body and mind.

Chapter 5

How the Mind
Affects the Body

Y OU ARE WALKING on a pure sandy beach with someone
you love. There is no one else on the beach. The sun is setting
in luminous bands of color. The sky is cloudless. Time is
forgotten. The moment is as lasting as the ocean itself, and as
intimate as the water that laps gently at your feet. Right now,
you haven't a care in the world.

When you concentrate on it for five to fifteen minutes a day,
this image and others like it can lower your blood pressure,
reduce and help control your cholesterol level, hormonal
imbalances, headaches, nervous tension, and strengthen your
body's ability to fight disease. It is called positive imaging, or
guided imagery, and it is a way to use the power of your mind
to control the inner environment of your body.

It is widely understood that the mind and body greatly
influence each other, and that strictly emotional and psychological factors can be the difference between health and
illness.

Sources for the information discussed and quotations cited in this chapter
are provided in the annotated bibliography.

Scientific evidence has demonstrated that one's emotions greatly affect the body's immune system, our major defense against disease. Positive feelings such as love, security, job satisfaction, and faith appear to strengthen the immune response, making it possible for the body to prevent and fight off illness. On the other hand, negative feelings, like excessive tension, worry, loss of hope, and depression, tend to weaken the immune response, sometimes to the point that it can be rendered helpless against an illness. Such emotional states have been linked to heart and artery diseases, cancer, lung ailments, kidney disorders, migraine headaches, diabetes, cirrhosis of the liver, suicide, and accidental injuries.

This means that your state of mind can crucially affect your health. It also means that with the right mental attitude you can, in a matter of weeks, learn to influence your inner responses and strengthen your body's immunity against disease.

To put it simply, the immune system attacks and destroys infection or aberrant cells in the body by marshaling antibodies — white blood cells or lymphocytes — that can destroy them. The white pus in a cut is nothing more than a collection of white blood cells that gather in the area to fight infection. During most of our lives, our immune systems are sufficiently powerful to eradicate most illnesses, or at least keep them in check so we can go on living, despite any problems that may be going on within us.

Until recently, medicine treated the mind and body as separate entities. Disease was believed to arise from a malfunction of the body. The way to treat disease, according to this view, was to correct the body deficiencies through the use of drugs and, to a lesser extent, surgery and radiation. The so-called wonder drugs, penicillin and the antibiotics, became the answer for every ailment.

When technology and pharmacology became pre-eminent, the physician's role as healer became less important than that of scientist or technician. In the role of technician the doctor tended to concentrate his or her attention on an individual organ — let's say the heart or gall bladder — or a particular symptom and its probable cause. The patient's attitude or state of mind was considered irrelevant to the healing process.

However, recent studies conducted on the subject leave little doubt that the mind can both reduce and enhance the effectiveness of the immune system. Mice have been found to contract cancer rapidly and in great numbers when they are placed under high levels of stress from noise, odor, and distress sounds from other animals, very much like the kinds of stressful stimuli many of us are subject to daily. However, when the same types of mice are provided with more comfortable living conditions, they experience less than 10 percent of the cancer rate suffered by the high-stress group.

Studies have shown that shocks administered to animals once every sixty seconds for only one hour shorten the time it takes for tumors to develop, increase the size of the tumors, and decrease the length of time the animals can survive once they have contracted the cancer. Other studies have demonstrated that the immune response can be conditioned to turn on and off simply by manipulation of the environment and emotional factors.

People who are highly goal oriented, workaholics, and driven by deadlines and ambition, typically referred to as type A individuals, have a far greater mortality rate from heart attack and stroke than other members of society. As a group, type A people suffer from higher-than-average blood pressure and heartbeat rate; they also show higher blood levels of such hormones as adrenalin, hydrocortisone, and insulin, all of which rise during times of stress.

When not dealt with effectively, prolonged stress results in hopelessness and despair, a sense that life contains little or no satisfaction. This occurs because the natural response to stress, the so-called flight-or-fight reaction, is suppressed, giving one the sense of being trapped, with no escape from the pressures of life. This only magnifies the stressful effects, and as researchers have discovered, often leads to some type of personal trauma, like divorce or midlife crisis. Researchers have found that such mental states also lead to illness and even death. Studies have shown that depression is the most common emotional condition preceding the onset of cancer.

In studying the effects of bereavement on those who had recently suffered the loss of a spouse, scientists discovered that the basic unit of the immune system, called a lymphocyte, failed to respond properly to disease. The lymphocyte did not activate against the illness, thus allowing the disease to spread. Bereavement, a wholly emotional state, had a deadening effect on the immune system.

Ultimately, stress is harmful to overall health in two ways: it creates the conditions within the body that themselves give rise to disease (elevating cholesterol levels, creating hormonal imbalances, and harming various organs), at the same time depressing the body's ability to fight illness by weakening the immune system.

These discoveries may provide some insight into why only a percentage of those who smoke get lung cancer, or why only some people exposed to a virus or a contagious disease become ill. Aside from the fact that some people eat better and follow sounder health habits, the level of stress is simply not the same in everyone's life; nor does everyone cope with stress with equal effectiveness. All of us develop cancer cells within our systems from time to time. Under normal conditions, the immune system is able to destroy these cells before they spread. However, the person who suffers from high levels of stress, and whose immune system is depressed as a result, may well be unable to destroy such aberrant cells, therefore permitting the malignancy to spread.

Take a moment to reflect on your own experiences with illness. Ask yourself what your emotional, psychological, and vocational states were like before you became sick, whether with a severe illness or simply a common cold.

In my own case, there was a distinctive pattern of mental and emotional reactions that can be charted, like points on a map, proceeding from my early forties, to the time I was diagnosed as having cancer at forty-seven, through the treatment period, and throughout my recovery.

Well before my disease was diagnosed, I suffered from a great deal of stress. In May 1978, Methodist Hospital was preparing for a major inspection by the Pennsylvania Department of Health, and as chief executive officer (CEO) I was responsible for seeing that the hospital was running at peak efficiency. The inspection was scheduled for the first week in June, and throughout the month of May I was overworked and anxious. Because I had only recently been appointed CEO of Methodist, some of the key staff and members of the hospital board of trustees still had doubts about my qualifications as a capable administrator. I understood that the outcome of the inspection would be reflected dramatically in my career. Thoughts of possible failure induced enormous tension in me.

In my early forties I had entered a midlife crisis that had a great deal to do with my lack of job satisfaction. I had been practicing anesthesiology for two decades, and the challenges and surprises of the job were gone. My career was my life, and when the luster went out of my job, it affected my entire existence. I found my solution in hospital administration — an entirely new career, full of new challenges and potential rewards. Any thought of having to give up my new profession and resume a job I thought I had outgrown sent a bolt of fear throughout my entire system. So the inspection became a kind of trial for me.

While I was preparing for the inspection, my father was dying of cancer. He lingered for about nine months, during which time my mother and I tried to keep him as comfortable as possible.

All of this—the inspection, the pressures of career and personal life, and my father's illness—seemed to converge on me, and then, on May 31, 1978, I too was told I had cancer.

It seems significant that once the diagnosis was made my back pain inexplicably became worse; when my father died in August and my last remaining hopes ran out, the pain and the symptoms of the disease became more intense.

Following the three operations I underwent and a short recovery period in the hospital, I was sent home to recuperate. There in the solitude of my apartment, my depression deepened. Thoughts of suicide were as close as my terrace railing, which, at twenty-seven floors up, would have provided an effective exit from my world of cancer and pain. Instead, I chose to go back to work, recognizing that if I did not do something to occupy my mind I would soon lose my weakening grip on sanity. There were still challenges to face on the job. These duties became important distractions from my world of self-pity and thoughts of death. They gave me something to live for. I was still a functioning human being who could make a contribution to his place of employment and to those around him. This provided me with a renewed sense of self-worth and inner strength. By going back to work I forced myself to recognize that I was quite capable of taking care of myself, and that I still had a great deal of strength left in my body and mind.

That insight was one of the early signs that my will to live was beginning to surface. I started to cope with my problem. I was willing to fight for my life. When an alternative presented itself, I was willing to gamble on a long shot and do my best to make it work.

My experience has taught me that once people commit themselves to the fight, they call on forces and strengths within that would not otherwise rally. The simple act of struggling against the odds is enough to kindle hope. We all have greater strengths than we realize, and once we have hope, we become resourceful. Positive emotions stimulate positive actions, which in turn bring about positive results. The evidence bears this out.

Dr. O. Carl Simonton, a radiation oncologist and a pioneer in the use of behavior and positive imagery in the treatment of cancer, has found that cancer patients with a positive attitude toward their chances of getting well fare far better and survive far longer than those who have a negative attitude about life and their therapy. Many of Simonton's patients report reversals of previously diagnosed incurable cancers.

In *Anatomy of an Illness,* Norman Cousins described his fight against a disease that affected the connective tissue of his body, for which doctors had no known treatment or cure. He was told that he had little, if any, chance of surviving. After hearing this verdict, Cousins took matters into his own hands. Working in conjunction with his doctor and immersing himself in the medical literature, he proceeded to develop his own recovery plan, which included such psychologically oriented therapies as laughter and the marshaling of affirmative emotions like love, faith, and hope. He also took large dosages of vitamin C, which, he concluded from his reading, would be helpful for his specific condition.

"It worked," Cousins wrote. "I made the joyous discovery that ten minutes of genuine belly laughter had an anesthetic effect and would give me at least two hours of pain-free sleep. When the pain-killing effect of the laughter wore off, we would switch on the motion picture projector again [he was watching Marx brothers films], and, not infrequently, it would lead to another pain-free interval."

Not only did laughter seem to help his sleep, but Cousins found that it also enhanced his body chemistry so that the inflammation from his disease actually decreased markedly several hours after each laughing episode.

Cousins went on to cure himself of his disease, despite his doctors' grim pronouncements that he would not survive. After turning his back on heavy medications, hospitals, and a death sentence, Cousins put what he learned from his experience succinctly: "Drugs are not always necessary. Belief in recovery always is."

The reason belief in recovery works is that belief enhances body chemistry and strengthens our ability to fight disease. Nowhere is this better demonstrated than in the study of placebos. A placebo is a substance that is made to look like medicine, but has no therapeutic value. More often than not, it is simply a sugar pill disguised as medication. However, research indicates that when a patient who is given a placebo for pain is told that it will provide pain relief, it very often does just that.

Researchers have found that placebos work not because people are fooling themselves into thinking that they are experiencing less pain, but because their brain chemistry is altered with their acceptance that a pill will bring about the desired effect. When a placebo is introduced, the brain secretes a group of substances called endorphins, which are morphinelike chemicals that have powerful pain-relieving qualities. They very often create a sense of well-being and mild euphoria. When a placebo is given, then another drug which can block the secretion of endorphins is administered, no pain relief will ensue, even if the patient believes that the placebo is a powerful analgesic. In other words, unless belief can be translated into a physiological reaction, the pain will remain constant. Thus, under normal circumstances, the body has the ability to turn belief into pain relief.

Brain chemistry is not the only function of the body affected by positive emotions. Blood cholesterol levels tend to be lowered with a reduction in tension and anxiety, and tension-induced hormonal imbalances tend to right themselves. With positive emotions, or belief, comes an overall reduction of stress and its attendant side effects, and with it a heightening of the body's ability to fight illness.

In a study at Ohio State University, researchers fed a population of rabbits a high-fat diet, which, as we pointed out in Chapter 2, raises blood cholesterol levels and increases the risk of heart attack and stroke. After a period of time, the rabbits were autopsied and their coronary arteries examined for atherosclerotic lesions (fat deposits clogging the arteries). All but a small subgroup of the rabbit population did in fact have coronary deposits. The researchers could not figure out why this smaller population—which had a 60 percent lower rate of coronary disease—escaped the effects of the high-fat diet. As it turned out, the smaller group of rabbits had been taken out of their cages every day and petted and talked to in loving tones by one of the researchers. Could the tenderness shown the rabbits be the reason one group turned out to be healthier?

The researchers decided to test the hypothesis and conducted the study twice more, each time taking a smaller group of rabbits out of their cages every day to stroke them and give them loving attention. The results of all three studies were the same. The rabbits that were treated with love and tenderness had far less atherosclerosis than the other test animals.

This phenomenon occurs in human populations as well. A remarkable example was studied in the township of Roseto, Pennsylvania, where residents experienced a surprisingly low incidence of heart attacks (one man per thousand died of a heart attack, while the national average is about 3.5 per thousand; Rosetan women were even further below the national norm). In addition, the Rosetans suffered from below-average rates of ulcers, senile dementia, and other common disorders. When researchers began to investigate the reasons behind these abnormally low levels of illness, they were amazed to find that a large percentage of the Rosetans suffered from obesity—a major risk factor in heart disease and other illnesses—and that their rates of high blood pressure and cholesterol levels were no different from those of the national norms, which is to say at high risk of illness. It was not surprising that investigators discovered that the Rosetan diet was typically rich in fat and other unhealthy constituents, and that the Rosetans did not exercise any more than the average American. Thus, the investigators ruled out physical activity as a factor in the Rosetans' low rates of disease.

What the researchers did find, however, was that Roseto was an extremely tightly knit community whose members regularly came to one another's aid in times of crisis. People in need routinely received food, money, and other assistance from family members and friends within the community. This kindness resulted in the enhanced ability of the Rosetans to cope with stress and ward off illnesses they might otherwise have to endure.

Our diet and exercise programs will help you reduce and control the stress in your life and make you better able to handle successfully the challenges with which life confronts you. But there is another highly effective method for controlling stress and developing a profound sense of peace, harmony, and faith in yourself. That method is meditation, or what some call guided imagery or prayer.

Meditation can reduce cholesterol levels and certain anxiety-producing hormones in the blood stream. It tends to induce deeper states of relaxation, reducing and eliminating tension, anxiety, and fear. Meditation creates in people who practice it a feeling of well-being that enhances their ability to have faith in themselves and their future. When you enter into a deep state of relaxation, the vicissitudes of life begin to fade away, like props on a stage. In meditation you experience a sense of timelessness, which helps you escape the cramped, trapped feeling that high anxiety tends to enforce on the psyche. You move beyond these limitations to a greater sense of peace. This is particularly true when you focus on positive images, such as the company and love of someone dear to you, or a place that you feel especially happy about.

Meditation can help people let go of long-standing conflicts with others, so that a feeling of reconciliation and forgiveness can replace resentment, rejection, or hatred. Some doctors speculate that just as negative emotions adversely affect certain areas of the brain, which in turn may suppress the immune function, positive emotions have the opposite effect—they stimulate the brain to enhance immune function. (We provide a series of meditation and guided imagery techniques in Chapter 7 to help you accomplish the goals discussed above.)

At first glance, meditation may appear to many as a rather ethereal practice, perhaps the stuff that dreams are made of, but laboratory tests show that such techniques improve our ability to handle stress, maintain good health, and overcome illness. Dr. Simonton points out that there is no such thing as a *spontaneous remission,* a term used by doctors to categorize a recovery that seems to have no cause. "In each case," he states, "there is some kind of cause-and-effect process. The process by which spontaneous remission takes place is simply beyond our present understanding." The same can be said for many of the unknown reasons that cause positive thoughts to have positive reactions on the body—we simply do not understand why such things work, only that in many cases they do.

Chapter 6

The Power of Faith

SO FAR WE HAVE LIMITED the discussion mostly to rational or scientifically based arguments for the health effects of sound diet, exercise, and the power of positive thinking, and, as you have seen, there is ample evidence to support the program outlined in this book. Yet there are times in our lives when rational thinking may not be enough. When my cancer was discovered, there was little science could do for me. Convinced that I would die if I did not resort to extraordinary means, I included as part of my therapy a program that, as far as I was concerned, had little or no scientific basis. In *Recalled by Life,* I described my introduction to a diet and philosophical system that ran counter to what I considered to be rational thought, and even common sense.

Since this was the only means of treatment I knew that offered me any real hope of surviving, it became clear that I would have to explore areas beyond the boundaries of science. In doing so, I was brought to a crisis that many of us face today, namely, how does one answer for oneself the deeper questions of life — questions of the spirit, of fate, and of the powers

Sources for the information discussed and quotations cited in this chapter are provided in the annotated bibliography.

that lie beyond our understanding—in the face of a society whose world view denies the existence of the spiritual or the supernatural? I also had to ask myself how one can believe in anything that science has yet to validate.

Let me share with you the story of my coming to have faith as a complement to my rational, intellectual perspective on life. In many ways, it is similar to that of other people who, when confronted with overwhelming obstacles, turned to God for strength and support and found both in abundance. This willingness to pray, or to believe that there is an infinite power to turn to, can't be accomplished all at once. In many cases, one has to literally change the way one thinks, which takes time and effort.

I had to learn to accept the fact that there are two ways of looking at reality: rationally, which says that everything in nature can be isolated as a separate and distinct entity whose movements are governed by an unconscious or mechanistic natural law; or spiritually, which points out that everything in nature, including all of life, is united, and that the movements of this entire unity are governed by a supreme force, or consciousness, whose goal is to bring everything into a higher state of being.

For most of my life I believed in the supremacy of rational thought and of science. It was not until I was confronted with my own mortality and with a philosophy that was antagonistic to rational thought that I began to see the limitations in my former views. Ironically, scientists working on the frontiers of physics, in a discipline called quantum mechanics, are demonstrating that all reality is indeed united and that matter and energy are but two manifestations of the same thing. This may require a considerable act of faith for many, but, as we shall see, the discoveries resulting from this advanced science have important spiritual implications.

Having faith in a supreme being or consciousness demands what may be a difficult intellectual commitment. The very way in which we have been taught to think is antagonistic to the idea of God, or to seeing reality as a unified whole. But perhaps with the help of science and traditional spiritual literature, we may be able to view reality in another way. The potential rewards from such a vision of reality can be victory over despair and doubt and relief from fear and pain during our darkest moments. A spiritual approach to life, for example, gives meaning to pain and shows the way to make some good come of our suffering.

I have come to believe that the force behind all existence, which I, like many others, call God, is infinitely loving and infinitely giving, but at the same time a ruthless taskmaster, a teacher who will literally stop at nothing to raise our consciousness. One of the ways he seems to do this is by confronting us with certain experiences that so baffle our sensibilities, so destroy our old beliefs, that we are brought to our knees like the rubble of a building that has collapsed. At this crucial point, a kind of rebirth, a transformation, can and often does take place: it is the start of a new life.

My story then is a shedding of old ideas through a series of very painful experiences and taking up new ways of being, which themselves will eventually grow old and have to be shed as well. The process continues until death.

We begin then with an idea that I held on to most firmly — that there was only one way of thinking, and that was rationally and scientifically. Like many educated Americans today, I once considered myself a supreme rationalist. For something to be thought of as true, it would have to demonstrate a physical presence. One could either experience the thing itself with one of the five senses or measure its effects with scientific instruments. In other words, everything that exists in nature reveals itself. That which doesn't reveal itself doesn't exist.

The basis for rationalist or naturalistic thinking was expounded by seventeenth-century mathematician and philosopher René Descartes, who foreshadowed the Enlightenment and argued that nature behaved in an orderly and systematic way. The universe, he said, worked like a great machine whose fundamental parts operated in a mechanical and predictable pattern, much like a clock. His view of the universe was mechanistic. He separated mind from matter, or the observer from the observed. He said that you could look at an event in nature without influencing or being influenced by it, just as if you were looking at a machine in operation.

The second part of Descartes's philosophy was that everything that occurred in the universe had a cause. Like reason itself, nature operated according to simple cause-and-effect relationships: *A* interacts with *B,* giving rise to *C.* Descartes's philosophy came to be known as the Cartesian world view.

The next giant who came into the picture was Isaac Newton, who provided the mathematical formulas that supported Descartes's philosophy. Newton showed that everything from the fall of an apple to the orbits of the planets operated according to orderly and systematic laws, which could be predicted mathematically, and, indeed, he succeeded in doing that. Newtonian physics provided the scientific basis for a mechanistic view of the universe, a view based on linear, or cause-and-effect, relationships.

The picture of the universe that emerged was something akin to a billiard game: one ball hits another, which in turn sets other balls in motion, ad infinitum. Every event in nature had an understandable cause. It was up to humanity to study nature to determine the causes that put various effects in motion.

Newtonian physics became the grandfather of all sciences; everything from medicine to psychology patterned itself after the Newtonian model. This was to become the rational answer for everything. The only appropriate way to discover the secrets of nature, in this view, was through an orderly and systematic approach, an approach that came to be known as the scientific method. Because it was based on Newtonian physics, the scientific method was used to isolate specific relationships to examine effects and their causes.

Enlightenment thinkers argued that because nature oper-
ates in orderly ways, miracles are impossible, since by
definition they violate the predictability and orderliness of
natural law. In the same way, questions of the supernatural, or
of God, were regarded as outside of reason, or of science. If
there were a God, he either could not or would not violate
natural law, and therefore could not participate in human
reality. Since no one could scientifically demonstrate the
presence of God, humanity was regarded as the center of the
universe, and, as such, human beings were left with the job of
unraveling and ultimately controlling nature's secrets.

The broadside against miracles and theism in general was
outlined most powerfully by the Enlightenment thinker David
Hume, whose essay "Of Miracles," published in the mid-
1700s, was so persuasive that it influenced both the educated
layperson and a great many of the clergy as well. From Hume's
day on, the laws of nature were thought of as inviolate, and
God or the supernatural became increasingly irrelevant.

It is easy to see that in such a philosophy, science and
technology were considered to be the only means by which
one could obtain knowledge. Because knowledge is fundamental to human survival, science acquired a godlike position
in society. In the same way, scientists themselves gained
power and prestige, while those who clung to religious beliefs,
including an all-powerful God, were looked upon as unsophis-
ticated, and even deluded.

Any doubts that this mechanistic view of the universe was
the only view were finally put to rest by two more Newtonian
thinkers—Charles Darwin and Sigmund Freud. In his *Origin
of Species* (1859), Darwin argued convincingly that life on earth
had gradually evolved over millions of years from a common
ancestry and that this evolution was accomplished through a
process called natural selection, or what later came to be
known as survival of the fittest. Since primordial times, living
things had been faced with the necessity of adapting to a

changing and hostile environment; those species that adapted by developing new characteristics, and were able to pass them on to their offspring, evolved and survived, while those that didn't disappeared. Though Darwin made a few perfunctory references to the Creator, his argument, for many, removed the necessity to consider God as the originator of life, and particularly as the creator of human beings. Darwin's agnosticism came to light in his 1871 book, *The Descent of Man;* after its publication his thoughts became a rallying point for the universal supremacy of humanity.

Finally, Freud's theories of the mind provided a basis for understanding human behavior. According to Freud, human psychology was shaped by the sexual nature of humanity and by relationships formed early in life, particularly those of the family. Freud viewed human beings as self-contained units who operated out of behavior patterns imprinted on them by their experiences. Here again we see the pre-eminence of cause-and-effect relationships. Every personality characteristic was manifested as a reaction to an external cause. God, Freud contended, was simply a projection of the father figure. As he once commented to Carl Jung, one of his most influential students, talk of the supernatural was "sheer bosh."

The important point here is that the scientific and intellectual establishment came to believe that human destiny was independent of divine intervention. Their science could find nothing beyond a law-abiding, mechanistic universe, which did not deviate from its orderly and predictable patterns. The human race appeared to be shaping its own future and would have to look to itself for salvation or oblivion. Moreover, if ever salvation were to come about, it would be by virtue of human reason and through its two most powerful instruments, science and technology.

I had adopted the Cartesian philosophy almost wholesale. By the time I entered college and medical school, Darwin and Freud were regarded as being above criticism. In the 1950s, although some might have argued with the specifics, Freudian psychology seemed to have a rational explanation for virtually every impulse in human behavior. After I became a doctor, my faith in science and technology became even stronger in view of medicine's ability to save lives and reestablish health. With the power of life and death seemingly in hand, humanity was, at the very least, the reigning power on earth, if not the center of the universe.

Nevertheless, despite the enormous power of rational thought, I still suspected that there might be more to life and human destiny than this naturalistic view of the universe. And yet, it made me uncomfortable to express such feelings even to myself. Every time people urged a more spiritual perspective on life, their arguments seemed more emotional than intellectual. As we all know, when it comes to providing a convincing argument, the heart is a rather blunt instrument, while the intellect has the cutting edge of a fine scalpel. The intellect is also a bloodthirsty adversary; it is wiser to keep one's spiritual yearnings quiet.

By the time I had graduated from medical school, my intellect had thoroughly controlled that part of me which hungered for spiritual fulfillment. I say *controlled,* not killed — the small voice within still spoke occasionally in a rather hushed, though haunting, whisper.

That whisper was never strong enough to stem my ambition for personal achievement and gratification, for rational thinking serves the ambitious well, and I was as ambitious as anyone. Since things exist as separate entities, and since there is no basis for spiritual reality, one has only to consider one's own priorities, which are usually ordered according to the single concern of survival. I fought to survive in the competitive realm of medicine and later in hospital administration. Since love requires a measure of selflessness, it obviously fails to thrive in highly competitive environments. Consequently, I found myself very much alone in the world, with a few close friends, some rather determined enemies, and little or no love. Ironically, at the very time when I had achieved my highest success — my appointment as chief executive officer at Methodist Hospital — I was confronted with my greatest life crisis — cancer. Suddenly, the whisper grew louder, and my gods of science and reason began to crumble.

In a sense, I had reached the limit of rational knowledge and power. I was about to die, and there was little medicine could do for me, except to remove a cancerous rib and my testicles. Despite the radical surgery and the drugs, my death seemed certain and imminent.

I was emotionally and spiritually crushed by the operations. I was a member of the Unitarian Church at the time; a Unitarian minister visited me daily while I was in the hospital and regularly while I recuperated at home. In the most kind and loving ways, he would ask me to reach out beyond myself for help and strength. But as a rationalist, I had absolutely no basis to believe in such things, especially now, as I lay broken in my bed. I was bitter. The profession to which I had dedicated my life could do nothing for me, and talk of a benevolent and giving God seemed like a cruel joke. How could such a God leave me in this state? Then I realized that my bitterness stood in the way of any chance I had of recovering, since it was an indulgence in self-pity, which is a consuming and weakening pastime.

Eventually, I wandered into a system that had no rational basis, but I clung to it because it offered me hope. In sticking with it, I was flung from my rational world into a metaphorical and mystical one. Indeed, the very way in which I was introduced to this foreign system was, in Jung's words, a most "meaningful coincidence."

On August 9, 1978, the day of my father's funeral, I was traveling south on the New Jersey Turnpike from the funeral grounds to my home in Philadelphia. Depressed and enduring raging back pain, I picked up two young hitchhikers, something that was highly uncharacteristic for me. They looked as though they were fresh out of college but I later learned that they had just graduated from a natural food cooking school in Boston. After some polite conversation, I mentioned to the young man sitting next to me that I was dying of cancer and that I had just buried my father, who had died of the same disease. This young cook — twenty-five years my junior — told me, in the most cavalier fashion, that I did not have to die, but that I could save myself by changing my diet and lifestyle.

Of course, at first I no more believed him than if he had told me he could fly. But the hook was in me. I didn't know it then, but I was already on the road to recovery. Within a month I was eating brown rice, vegetables, and seaweed in a commune and trying desperately, but skeptically, to get well.

Throughout the course of my recovery, I was exposed to methods of healing, diet and acupuncture being the two most important, of which Western medicine has no appreciation. There were no acceptable studies to prove that acupuncture had any real therapeutic value; it simply did not exist as far as Western medicine was concerned. And the studies showing diet to be useful in preventing cancer, heart disease, and other illnesses were just coming to light and were still the subject of enormous controversy. Even so, no one claimed that nutrition could be a factor in the treatment of cancer.

As I watched myself get better, however, I increasingly came to believe in the power of these methods. What rattled my rational foundation all the more was the fact that diet and acupuncture (and acupressure massage, or Do-In) were explained in terms that were antithetical to rational thought. But that only stood to reason, since these disciplines were three thousand years old; such methods had been developed in the ancient world, long before our current brand of rational thinking assumed its dominant place in the human mind.

As stated in Chapter 4, the explanation for acupuncture involves the presence of a universal energy, called *ki* or *prana* in the East, which is believed to exist in all living things and is regarded as the very fuel of life. Diet and acupuncture merely enhance the flow of energy, bringing the body into a state of balance, or into a state whereby this energy flows through the body unimpeded. Other behavior patterns can also influence this flow of energy. Anger, fear, and tension, for example, tend to block or trap energy in various parts of the body, giving rise to illness, while laughter, joy, and love allow energy to flow naturally from the body to the person or thing that evokes the response.

To a Westerner, this explanation sounded more like theology than science. A universal source of energy that was the very source of life seemed like another way of talking about God and his grace. Whether we called it *ki* or grace didn't seem to matter; what mattered was that although it was difficult, if not impossible, to make sense of this system from a scientific point of view, it made good sense from a theological perspective. Could this energy field that surrounded the body, according to these Easterners, in fact be the human soul? Certainly, an energy field that gave the body life need not die when the body ceases to exist. Energy does not depend on oxygen, or any other biological life-support system, for its existence. Indeed, energy exists in all forms of matter throughout the universe. Couldn't this energy field, or the consciousness we call the soul, simply move on to another state of being?

Such speculations gave a dreamlike quality to my life and provided the basis for my severe internal conflict. I was continually at war with myself. What I was hearing was an Eastern interpretation of God and his infinite power. Indeed, the only way I was ever going to recover, according to this view, was by opening up myself to this healing energy, or grace. My rational mind could not tolerate such concepts as *ki*, or even dietary therapy, for that matter; meanwhile, the hushed voice within was growing more bold — it desperately wanted to believe. And my life hung in the balance.

Still, my acceptance of this point of view was made more difficult by the Oriental or Eastern perception of reality, a view that diametrically opposes rational thought. While a rationalist sees reality as an interaction of objects moving in space, the Oriental perceives reality as a single picture, with all its elements united and interdependent. Every element in the picture is a vital necessity to the completeness of the whole. As a result, nothing can be separated or isolated without altering, indeed falsifying, the integrity of the picture, or one's perception of reality. This is essentially the holistic, or monistic, perspective, which says that every single event in the universe is related to, and dependent on, every other event, no matter how far apart any two may appear to be. Thus, the observer and the observed are united in the moment they experience together, each influencing the other, since both are part of the larger picture, or single event, called the universe.

This philosophy was really saying that the very universe itself is one great living being, and that every single event or object in the universe can be likened to an individual function or cell within a gigantic living body. The universe is one. While a cell within your body can be thought of as separate and distinct, it nonetheless depends on the body as a whole, and all the living systems within the body, for its life. The body, too, depends on its cells, both collectively and individually, for its life. One does not exist without the other. In the same way, whatever happens anywhere in the cosmos has an impact on me, and I on it, since I am part of this larger body, this living entity we call reality.

Throughout the winter of 1978 and the spring and summer of 1979, I took my meals with a family who proselytized Eastern dietary and philosophical thought. I joined several other students and family members each night to share this strange diet and talk about such esoteric and abstruse subjects as the health effects of diet, Oriental philosophy, some of the great Eastern philosophical works, the philosophy of yin and yang, and the holistic vision of reality.

In the early going, I was certain I had plunged myself

directly into madness. Each night I would go home from dinner and wonder whether I was losing my grip on sanity. I felt a great conflict because the philosophy appealed to an aesthetic, perhaps spiritual, part of me. Certainly one had to be selective about how much of these views one should swallow; there was a lot of chaff among the wheat. Still, the spiritual perspective gave me a sense of having a great deal more power and authority within me than the rational perspective could ever provide. After all, the spiritual approach argued that I had the power of the universe on my side and that I was connected to an infinite supply of energy. All I had to do was draw on this limitless account by maintaining healthy eating habits, exercise, and prayer or meditation. The mystics of both East and West made the same claim; through fasting, prayer, and a simple lifestyle, one purified oneself. One became a clearer vessel for the subtle inspiration of God. One's actions took on more meaning because they were motivated by higher spiritual forces rather than the capricious impulses of the appetites.

Unfortunately, I did not live and work in a monastery in Tibet, but in a high-rise apartment building in downtown Philadelphia. What was fine in Tibet somehow didn't translate to South Broad Street. I had only to wake up in the morning and go off to my office to know just how far I had traveled from the world in which I had grown up.

Every day I crossed back and forth between these two worlds — from the Cartesian world view, which was the basis of modern medicine, to the holistic vision of reality, which was the foundation of the diet and philosophy that I hoped would help save my life. Needless to say, I suffered from something of an identity crisis. There was nothing in my background to help me cope with a new way of thinking, other than my childhood exposure to Christian beliefs expounded by the Catholic Church. However, I had left the church many years ago, and its precepts were no longer part of my everyday consciousness. Indeed, this regime seemed so foreign to me that it appeared as if the people who were promoting it were inventing explanations for reality as they went along. Was there something to this spiritual, or holistic, view, or had I fallen into Wonderland?

I seemed to have two choices: either suspend my rational judgment and hope that there was value in what I was doing, or simply deny that there might be any substance in what was happening to me. I alternated between both.

Fortunately for my sanity, I underwent regular medical tests, which seemed to interject at least a familiar reality. The tests showed that my health was clearly improving. My foreign and unorthodox approach seemed to be working, either because or in spite of the metaphorical explanation that served as its basis.

Soon I began to question whether rational thinking was the only way to look at the universe, or to uncover its truths. The possibility that began to emerge was that rationalist thinking was true, as far as it went, but that there could be a complementary and opposite view of reality which might be equally true.

Certainly, the Newtonian model, as modern physicists were pointing out, had severe limitations. For one thing, the scientific method employed in the modern laboratory is equipped only to examine events that can be reproduced under specifically controlled conditions. Scientific studies in the traditional framework must be based on the examination of cause-and-effect relationships. Unique events, or those influenced by chance, are beyond the realm of science. Indeed, the laboratory setting attempts to exclude chance in order to examine the interaction of two or more factors in isolation. And yet, what situation in our lives is not influenced by chance or by circumstances that we could not have predicted?

As Jung wrote, "If we leave things to nature, we see a very

different picture [from that produced in the laboratory]: every process is partially or totally interfered with by chance, so much so that under natural circumstances a course of events absolutely conforming to specific laws is almost an exception."

Chance is so much a part of our lives that virtually all of us recognize our vulnerability to chance occurrences. How many times, for example, have we felt the shadow of concern cross our minds when a loved one walks out the front door on an otherwise routine errand? We know that chance travels on the backs of both danger and deliverance. It is only through an equally undependable faculty we call intuition that chance occurrences can be foreseen, or "felt."

It is impossible to predict with any degree of certainty what will happen in any human life. Chance events take place every moment; the possibilities are endless. Chance is an important element in both contracting and recovering from illness.

The fact is that you and I are unique events in nature. No doctor can tell you what will happen to *you*, no matter what your state of health. A physician can tell you only what the statistical picture looks like. From a statistical point of view, the chances of my surviving my cancer were painfully slim, so slim that it appeared unlikely I would live for four years following the diagnosis of the disease. As long as I accepted the statistical outlook I should certainly have been given up for dead. But each of us is a unique entity in the universe, subject to unique and unpredictable occurrences. Science could not predict that I would meet two hitchhikers on the New Jersey Turnpike, that I would begin eating a grain and vegetable diet, that I would pray regularly, and that I would experience a remarkable recovery of my health.

In September 1979, I scheduled a bone scan to discover how much progress I had made. Just before the test, one of my physicians explained to me that he expected to find the disease in the same pattern it had been in fourteen months earlier. He was optimistic that I had arrested the disease, but he expected the cancerous lesions to continue to be spread throughout my body. He cautioned me not to expect much change; bones take a long time to heal, I was told.

The tests showed that I was completely free of cancer; there were no lesions anywhere in my body; my bones had healed.

Naturally, this was far more than anything I had expected. Somehow many factors had come together to bring about this unusual, if not unique, event. Certainly I had contributed to the process of getting well by following an excellent diet and exercise program; I had encouraged my immune system to make a fight of it. But the mechanism by which these components came together in proper measure was, for me, miraculous.

At this point in my life I had begun to open up to the possibility of miracles. Too much had happened to me to simply close the door on such thoughts. Intellectually, I could see that unique events were always happening, and thus Hume stood corrected. If there were a God who wanted to participate in human reality, he could do it simply by choosing to alter the course of individual lives, and history, through the occurrence of what would appear to us to be a unique or chance event.

In the days that followed my bone scan, I felt like a modern-day Lazarus. I had returned from a long and dark stay in the grave. My new life, by contrast, was almost unbearably rich and joyful. I was imbued with an energy that reached beyond me, made me feel more powerful and alive than I'd ever felt before. That small voice within was now like the mouse that roared; it urged me on to a place where it could fully express itself.

For reasons not entirely clear to me, I felt drawn to my religious roots in Roman Catholicism. Philadelphia's Cathedral of Saints Peter and Paul is a mammoth structure, nearly a city block in size, a place rich in mystery and intimations of the infinite. Inside its darkened recesses candles flicker like numinous beings of light. The seemingly endless rows of pews line up in a study in perspective, giving one a sense of the progression of time and space. Beyond the pews lies the altar — tall, ornate, and softly lighted under a marble canopy supported by four large marble columns. The high ceiling is carved and touched by gold leaf inlay. Tall, multicolored stained-glass windows throw a rainbow of hues down upon the polished marble floors, and in the air the smell of incense hangs like a warm and relaxing memory.

Whenever I entered the cathedral and let the big door shut behind me, I felt the noise and confusion of my life fade. The ceaseless and badgering complaints were dominated by the quiet solitude and peacefulness that reigned within this building. There was an overpowering sense of presence here, the feeling that some magnificent life had occupied and permeated this place.

In describing the human psyche (the "self"), Jung suggested that beyond the conscious and unconscious minds lies the collective unconscious — an infinite storehouse of information handed down from generation to generation since primordial times. The information and the images that came to us via the collective unconscious, images that Jung called archetypes, represented a knowledge developed from the whole of our ancestral past. As a result of this knowledge, certain relationships and events in the development of human consciousness are already partially understood. Among these archetypes are the images of mother and her many roles, the earth, birth, childhood, adulthood, old age, certain fears (of the dark, of snakes, of falling, for example), and the image of God. None of these images has to be implanted in the newborn's mind through education or experience; all that needs to happen is for experience to fill in the details of the images, and in this way the archetypes give our lives direction; we seek from birth to experience them, to fill in the details, to solve the mysteries they present to us. In choosing to develop certain aspects of our personalities — certain archetypes — we determine what kinds of people we become.

Somehow this cathedral and its atmosphere, the Mass, and my own experiences in prayer seemed to bring forth a sense of these primordial archetypes, opening a door to a truly deep recess within me, a center of consciousness that was beyond me but also a part of me. As Jung pointed out, myth and religion are rich in these archetypal images. Such images provide the basis of the Catholic service: the communion; the promise of the Resurrection, or life after death; the eternal flame, signifying the limitlessness of life; the showering of blessings on those who maintained as best they could the pursuit of a higher ideal. In participating in the Mass, I took part in something ancient, healing, and continuous. There I experienced an exchange of psychic energy: my distress, my despair, my endless fears of pain and death were transformed to a degree of restfulness and a certain security; my focus went from my immediate needs to those of a longer-term agenda — the needs of my soul.

As Jung pointed out, every religion has its archetypal imagery, its language of the soul. There have always been the priests, rabbis, shamans, spiritual teachers, guides, and medicine men whose function in society is to interpret the signs of heaven and earth in the lives of individuals. These archetypes have remained relatively uniform throughout history, and they have been the basis for traditional religious ceremonies, myths, and rites of passage. The need to acknowledge a relationship with God and to the unity of reality, to all of humanity, springs from this eternal well, this collective unconscious. I had seen the importance and power of Eastern thought, and now the beauty and inspiration of the Judeo-Christian traditions were rekindled within me. Some powerful energy filled me in these rituals. I deeply believe that all of this was fundamental to my recovery and the maintenance of my health.

Yet, when I left the peacefulness and splendor of this fine church, I still had not resolved the rational and religious or mystical perspectives — paradoxical and seemingly contradictory ways of looking at reality—that existed within me in a very tenuous balance. Once the elation of my recovery wore off, I needed to make sense of my cancer and the pain that had resulted. By the fall of 1979, I was spending hours in the library, attempting to find clues that might provide an intellectual basis for what had happened to me.

Almost instantly, I found an abundance of recent scientific evidence linking diet to disease. My introduction to a diet of whole grains and vegetables was based solely on faith in a system that was apparently inexplicable from a rational point of view. I found that science supported, at least in part, what the spiritual perspective recommended in diet.

I was hoping to find a scientific basis for the wider, more spiritual reality I was experiencing. Was there really something to this spiritual view of reality that seemed to extend so far beyond Newtonian physics? The answer was in quantum mechanics, recognized today as our most advanced science on the nature of the universe. Quantum mechanics has demonstrated that the reality of the universe is a lot more complicated than the Newtonian world that we perceive with our five senses, and far more difficult to understand; that change occurs casually and randomly and, often, seemingly of its own accord; that the observer and the observed event cannot be separated, since they interact mutually and affect each other; that matter itself, the very stuff that makes up our bodies and our entire physical universe, behaves paradoxically: it is orderly and predictable (as Newton had said), but also disorderly and unpredictable. In other words, matter does not behave logically.

"The universe can appear to be both fundamentally paradoxical, chaotic, and indeterminant, and, at the same time, logical, orderly, and quite determinate," wrote quantum physicist Fred Alan Wolf in *Taking the Quantum Leap*. The only way to resolve the paradox, he points out, is for the observer to choose whichever reality he or she prefers. Both are correct, yet each is an incomplete view of reality without the other.

Matter, the very basis of what most of us take to be real and predictable, behaves as if it were composed of both physical particles (that is, atoms) and nonphysical waves. When the physicist attempts to conduct an experiment to determine which is the dominant presence (particles or waves), it turns out to be both — that is, particles that behave as expected up to a point, then suddenly change into waves without warning.

Wolf discussed an experiment physicists perform to find out whether the basic building block of a pencil is particle or wave. Atomic physicists, he wrote, "see the pencil as atomic particles, tiny points of substance, like little ball bearings or itsy-bitsy baseballs. Reality is to them, and probably to most of us, solid." However, when the physicist breaks down the pencil into its component parts, he finds that those fundamental parts do unpredictable things. "The little baseballs do not behave like little baseballs — they diffract or bend and spread out like waves, producing wave patterns when collected together and individual marks when seen separately."

So physicists have trouble deciding what actually makes up a pencil, or a tree, or a human being, or all the matter in the universe: particles or waves, that is, solid points of substance or ever-moving waves.

Two thoughts that supersede Newtonian physics are implicit here: the first is that reality is composed of paradoxical phenomena — it is orderly yet unpredictable. "Nature is dualistic," wrote Wolf. "There was always a hidden, complementary side to everything that we experienced ... The more we determine one side of reality, the less the other side is shown to us."

Newton and other Enlightenment thinkers developed their views according to the orderly side of nature, and thus they were prevented from seeing that order was continually being complemented by the unpredictable or chance event. Such Enlightenment thinkers as Hume argued that miracles could never occur because nothing could violate the orderliness of natural law. Quantum physics has proved otherwise, and we see an agency through which miracles can occur.

The second part of the particle-wave revelation is that the observer and the observed event influence each other; in other words, reality is a subjective phenomenon, created — at least in part — by the observer himself. As observers of any event, we influence the event by our presence, our thoughts, and our prejudices; further, we also shape our own perceptions of the event by noticing certain aspects that occur, failing to notice others, and reacting to the event in a unique way, making objectivity impossible.

"Quantum physics has taught us that we, the observers of reality, are, at the same time, the participants in reality," said Wolf. "In other words, 'observation' is not a passive noun; 'to observe' is not a passive verb ... objectivity is only an illusion."

We participate in, not merely witness, all the events we observe in our lives. For example, the minute I walk onto a field of grass, I begin to interact with the field — it affects my senses, it changes my inner reality, it alters my state of consciousness. I, in turn, change the nature of the field by leaving my footprints in its soil. Furthermore, I am in effect creating this meadow by my ability or inability to observe it. Those things I fail to observe never exist for me. Perhaps I am worried or sad or have other thoughts on my mind that clutter my consciousness, further blocking my awareness; the reality of this grassy field is diminished all the more. Or perhaps the opposite is true: my thoughts are entirely directed at the beauty of the grassy field; I have positive associations with such places, and these feelings fill my inner reality. I bend down to smell a flower, or notice the way the wind blows the grass in an easterly direction. I feel the wind and sun on my cheeks. I love this place and the feelings it has inspired in me. I am happy.

The field and I relate on other levels as well. I breathe in billions of atoms of oxygen that have been produced by the grass; it breathes in millions of molecules of carbon dioxide that I breathe out. I affect the way the sun and wind hit the grass; perhaps I've frightened away a few animals that might feed on the grass and other plants here. It is no longer an empty meadow, but a field with a man standing in the middle of it. I have changed this place, and it has changed me.

My experience of the field is purely subjective, as are all my experiences. As we have seen, even the laboratory setting, which goes to great lengths to control the environment, excludes phenomena that might otherwise occur in nature, thus making the laboratory setting a creation of subjective views of reality, as well.

This interaction is even more profound on the atomic level, where quantum physicists have found that every time they attempt to look at an atom, they alter its behavior and position dramatically. The picture of atoms scientists have found is at least partially created by their very act of looking. Physicists have begun to wonder if atoms exist at all, or at least if they do before scientists actually look for them.

Contrary to what Newton said, there are no objective perceptions of the universe; one cannot separate oneself from events in nature and expect to get a correct or complete view of those events. Wolf said,

> We are actively choosing the reality of the world each instant, and during the same instant, we are unaware that we are doing it. But our becoming aware of this simple truth can enable us to see the world's complementary side. And once we see this complementary side of reality, our old prejudices ... will crumble. The barriers that separate mind and matter will dissolve. God and human will reconcile.

These and other scientific discoveries have given rise to an entirely new view of reality, which is not Newtonian. Quantum physicist Fritjof Capra, author of *The Tao of Physics,* said,

> The shift is toward a world view that you can call a holistic view, or an organic view, an ecological view ... Ecological because it is characterized by the notion of the fundamental inter-

dependence between all phenomena ... As Neils Bohr emphasized, the main consequence of these theories was that you could not separate any part of the material universe from the rest without making an error ... The new vision of reality is a spiritual vision in its very essence ... The human spirit, as I've come to see it, is the mode of consciousness in which the individual becomes aware of being connected to the cosmos as a whole. The mode of consciousness is much broader than a rational mode, it is an intuitive mode. It typically occurs in meditative experiences but can also occur in many other settings.

Such a view of reality has enormous implications for human behavior. By our thoughts and prejudices we perceive the world and create it within us. By our actions, based on those perceptions, we send out infinite ripples into a sea of oneness. Positive thoughts and actions can transform the world into a positive place to be; negative thoughts create a negative world. Each of us re-creates the world in his or her own image. As individuals, and as a collective society, we are responsible for the state of the world as we perceive it. This, of course, has a very practical application for health.

In Chapter 5 we showed that our thoughts can directly affect our health. Positive thoughts about ourselves and others, such as loving support from friends and family, appear to be health-promoting. On the other hand, negative thoughts and antagonistic relationships, feelings of being alone or separated, all have a negative effect on health. Here we see quantum theory applied to our lives. Thoughts and actions that are in line with the universe, that unite us with others, have a health-promoting effect. In order to unite, we must establish the well-being of others as a priority in our lives — in other words, we must learn to love one another. Human experience has shown us that love is the unifying force in the world, and most probably in the universe itself. Actions that separate us from others, although theoretically impossible in light of quantum reality, seem to go against something basic in the universe, indeed in ourselves, and thus are physically debilitating.

The idea of a living, spiritual, holistic universe is fundamental to the spiritual teachings of both West and East. "Hear, O Israel: The Lord our God, the Lord is One" and "Love thy neighbour as thyself" are two of the most important thoughts in spiritual life.

It is through the One that all things are brought into being. In the *Tao Te Ching,* the seminal work that forms the basis of Taoism, one of the most important religions in the history of China and the Orient in general, Lao-tzu writes that the One is both the giver of life and the benefactor of wisdom.

> These things in ancient times received the One:
> The sky obtained it and was clarified;
> The earth received it and was settled firm;
> The spirits got it and were energized;
> The valleys had it, filled to overflow;
> All things, as they partook it came alive;
> The nobles and the king imbibed the One
> In order that the realm might upright be;
> Such things were then accomplished by the One ...
> Truly, a cart is more than the sum of its parts.

This passage, of course, is reminiscent of Genesis, which begins, "In the beginning God created the heaven and the earth." The last line of Lao-tzu's poem takes the point a step further. God is not only the creator of life, but he is greater than the sum of his creations; God's consciousness extends beyond that which he has made.

That the whole is greater than the sum of its parts is true in our own experience as well as in quantum mechanics. This represents another break with Descartes and Newton, both of whom thought that the whole was no more than the actions of its individual parts, a premise on which modern Western medicine and most other sciences are founded.

But perhaps quantum theory offers yet another key to understanding spiritual realities, and particularly the evolution of consciousness. That key is the idea of paradox. Quantum mechanics points out that all things are composed of complementary and contradictory sides—both particles and waves, or order and chance, for example. Traditional spiritual literature maintained the same view: that one state of being changes into its opposite. The Chinese called this complementary and antagonistic relationship yin and yang. Heraclitus and other Greek philosophers recognized it as the paradoxical state of being. For both the Greeks and the Chinese, all things were brought into existence by the interaction of opposing tendencies, which at first clash and then reconcile to produce the new birth. For example, a single twenty-four-hour period is composed of both day and night, or light and dark; temperature is differentiated by the existence of hot and cold; growth and decay are made possible through the processes of expansion and contraction; stature is differentiated between high and low; man and woman are necessary to bring forth human life. In short, things are brought into being by the presence of their complementary opposites, which naturally appear antagonistic at first because their qualities are different. Yet an experience that is antagonistic to us forces us to change; when it is complementary, it fulfills us, or aids us in becoming more than what we presently are.

Heraclitus wrote, "Opposition brings concord. Out of discord comes the fairest harmony . . . It is by disease that health is pleasant, by evil that good is pleasant, by hunger satiety, by weariness rest."

I have come to believe that my cancer, and all the difficulties I faced following the onset of the disease, was antagonistic to my former ways of being, yet complementary in that it gave me a new way of looking at life. Because I was extremely intractable and bent on self-gratification on all levels, I needed a powerful stimulant to grow. My cancer, as it turned out, served that purpose. Many people have been transformed in fundamental ways by an experience that brought them to the precipice of death. I was no different. When I was preparing to die, I was hopelessly alone in the world. By the time my life was restored, I knew how to be different and make my existence worthwhile.

In this context suffering takes on a new and meaningful significance. Viewed in this light, suffering can be the first step toward the attainment of its opposite, which is peace.

In *Answer to Job,* Jung explored the duality and paradoxical nature of suffering as it is employed by God. According to Jung, Job is raised to a state of enlightenment by virtue of his suffering — inflicted on him by God himself — and by the fact that Job behaves correctly in the face of his adversity.

The story opens with Job a wealthy landowner, the proud father of ten children, and the employer of many servants. His life is rich and full, and because he is a faithful and religious man he is fervent in his expressions of gratitude to God. Suddenly, however, he is robbed of all his wealth, suffers the death of his children and servants, and is made to endure a plague of boils on his flesh when God is persuaded by Satan to test Job's faithfulness. In the metaphor of this fable, God allows ill fate to befall Job, when he could just as easily have consulted his own omniscience to discover whether or not Job is a faithful steward of the Lord. Instead, he allows treachery to invade Job's life.

Job's reaction is truly extraordinary. He says: "Naked came I out of my mother's womb, and naked shall I return thither: the Lord gave and the Lord hath taken away; blessed be the name of the Lord." (Job 1:21)

In the blink of an eye, Job goes from being blessed with a large family, wealth, and many servants to a poor and humble man all alone. It is as if, having enjoyed the richness of the daytime, in which the sun had showered down its blessings on his land, he suddenly was doomed to the cold and lifeless night. He is made to suffer the antithesis of his happiness and wealth.

Remarkably, Job remains unshaken in his faith; he recognizes that God is One, and thus understands who has brought down such cruel and unusual punishment on him. Yet he does not see this as a reason to stoop to anything but correct moral behavior. He continues to pray to God to be restored to his former state, knowing all the while that there also exists within God an advocate for humanity to whom he can appeal for help. Job sees God's use of paradox; God confronts Job with experiences that baffle him and bring him pain. Then he sits back and observes Job's reactions.

For what end is Job made to experience such cruel and seemingly unwarranted treatment?

Jung wrote, "We must . . . keep an eye on the background of all these events. It is just possible that something in this background will gradually begin to take shape as compensation for Job's undeserved suffering."

That compensation comes in the gift of wisdom. In refusing to give in to anything but correct moral behavior, Job represents a moral force in the world, a beacon of faith. He sets his life on principles that are bigger than he is, that go beyond him, that are themselves archetypes of virtue. Job embodies these virtues, makes them his own, and in so doing ascends to a place of honor and wisdom equal to them. Job possesses characteristics that he did not possess before his trials began. He has enriched his character by enduring in correct behavior in the face of enormous difficulties. Job comes to understand God's uses of difficulties to strengthen character and raise one's level of consciousness.

"The tortured though guiltless Job has secretly been lifted up to a superior knowledge of God," wrote Jung. Job realizes

God's use of paradox for the evolution of the soul, and in light of this realization his knowledge attains a divine wisdom.

In coming to understand God's paradoxical acts, Job gains insight into God's infinite power. For just as opposite sexes are required within humanity to produce life, so does God rely on opposites within himself to bring forth creation and the evolution of the spirit.

"Yahweh is not a human being: he is both persecutor and helper in one, and the one aspect is as real as the other," wrote Jung.

In attaining his divine wisdom, Job is granted an audience with the Lord, after which he is restored to his former happiness and wealth. Through his suffering, Job has attained wisdom. He "has learnt his lesson well and experienced 'wonderful things' which are none too easily grasped," Jung remarked. Thus, Job's trials take on illuminating significance.

The message in the story of Job is carried throughout the New Testament and the teachings of Christ, for so much that comes after Job seems to be illuminated in light of Job's discovery: that one life condition often turns into its opposite for the evolution of consciousness, or of the soul. The teachings of Jesus are replete with such a message.

But many that are first shall be last; and the last shall be first. (Matt. 19:30)

And whosoever shall exalt himself shall be abased; and he that shall humble himself shall be exalted. (Matt. 23:12)

Blessed are the poor in spirit: for theirs is the kingdom of heaven.
     Blessed are they that mourn: for they shall be comforted.
     Blessed are the meek: for they shall inherit the earth.
     Blessed are they which do hunger and thirst after righteousness: for they shall be filled. (Matt. 5:3–6)

Blessed are they which are persecuted for righteousness' sake: for theirs is the kingdom of heaven. (Matt. 5:10)

The spiritual literature of the East is equally rich with such a message. In the *Tao Te Ching,* Lao-tzu provides almost the same message as Jesus' Sermon on the Mount:

> The crooked shall be made straight
> And the rough places plain;
> The pools shall be filled
> And the worn renewed;
> The needy shall receive
> And the rich shall be perplexed.

Perhaps difficulties, when they evoke appropriate responses, precede revelation. I had never reflected so much on my own life, or made so many important changes, as when I got cancer. Like Job, I cursed my life when my trials began; unlike Job, I did not respond with great faith. On the contrary, I had to be convinced, or even coerced, into believing. But in the end, believing saved us both.

Chapter 7

Exercises for Peace of Mind

So MUCH for the theory of meditation and spiritual enlightenment; now let's get down to practical realities. Perhaps you've had a rough day at the office or your children are pushing you to the breaking point. Your nerves are as taut as piano wire, and your stomach is so acidic that it feels as if it's being electrocuted. Your impulse may be to scream or grab a double scotch, or both, but there is another way. You can take the phone off the hook, go into a softly lighted room, and revel in a deep state of relaxation for fifteen minutes, after which you can emerge feeling renewed and alive again. In so short a period, you can restore balance to your body and mind while taking important steps toward improving your health and ability to fight disease. No drink or scream, however primal it may be, can do for you what fifteen minutes of deep relaxation can.

Relaxation is the natural way to reduce stress and eliminate its negative side effects. By mastering a few simple techniques,

Sources for the information discussed and quotations cited in this chapter are provided in the annotated bibliography.

you can create a state of relaxation whenever you want to and wherever you are. The exercises described below will teach you how to control and overcome nervous tension, anxiety, and fear. They will help you achieve a deep state of relaxation in minutes, creating within you a sense of peace and well-being. They will help you control and overcome the negative side effects of stress. They are designed to help your body fight disease, as well as help you deal with external difficulties with the wisdom that comes from calmness and inner peace.

We have provided several types of short but highly effective meditation exercises, which are a sort of warm-up for the more elaborate guided imagery techniques that follow.

These exercises require only five to fifteen minutes each to be effective, although the longer you do them the more relaxed you become, and the more you allow the positive emotions and thoughts to become a part of you. We recommend that you do one of the suggested meditations — any one of the short exercises or the guided imagery techniques — three times a day. This amounts to a total of fifteen to forty-five minutes a day, depending on how long you wish to pursue each exercise. The more you do the exercises, the more they will become second nature to you, so that you will be able to use them during short periods of time in virtually any place you wish.

Before you begin your meditation, you should take some rudimentary steps to relax yourself. First, go to a softly lighted room and sit in a comfortable chair, preferably one with a straight back. Take off your shoes and sit back. Take note of your breathing. Is it rapid or slow, shallow or deep? Slow down your breathing and draw your breath deep into your abdomen, so that your stomach swells with every inhalation. Breathe in and out very slowly, deeply, and naturally. Feel the tension draining from your body. Once you've done this, you'll be ready to begin one of the meditation techniques described below.

The Short Meditative Exercises

Concentrate on a Word or a Short Passage

A particular word or a short passage has been used with great effectiveness to bring about deep states of relaxation and a sense of well-being. The idea is to focus on the word, called a mantra in the East, or a short passage by repeating it over and over again in your mind in a slow, rhythmic fashion until other thoughts and images are eliminated and positive feelings and associations well up inside you. The longer you focus on the word or phrase, the longer the good feelings that are inspired will stay with you, having a strengthening and health-promoting effect. Soon a peaceful, timeless quality settles over you. You are in a place removed from the world; your energies are restored, your batteries recharged.

If you have trouble focusing on a passage or word, you may want to chant the word or phrase softly to yourself. This creates a wonderful inner resonance and profound relaxation. Because you are using energy, you experience a deeper sense of release afterward.

Words that have been used as mantras for silent prayer or chanting include *shalom,* the Hebrew word for "peace"; *abba,* the ancient Hebrew word for "father" or "God"; the Sanskrit word *om* or *aum,* used in Oriental traditions to signify the universal sound; the names of a variety of spiritual and religious figures; and for some, their own names. This meditative device was used by Alfred Lord Tennyson and Walt Whitman, among others. In *Walt Whitman: A Life,* Justin Kaplan quoted Whitman as writing: "What am I after all but a child, pleas'd with the sound of my own name? repeating it over and over; I stand apart to hear — it never tires me." Whitman used the words *stand apart* to suggest the ecstatic spiritual experience such chanting brought on for him. The idea of chanting one's own name may sound somewhat egotistical to many, and it's obviously not for everyone, but it has been known to awaken parts of one's identity that were previously unknown or misunderstood. Whitman himself experienced a spiritual rebirth: "I cannot be awake," he wrote afterward, "for nothing looks to me as it did before. Or else I am awake for the first time, and all before has been a mean sleep." This spiritual awakening brought forth genius, and a literature that still stands as the poetic voice of America.

So many short passages in spiritual literature, music, and poetry can be used to recite in meditation that it would be impossible to create any short or representative list. A cursory review of the world's great religious books, including the Old and New Testaments, the *Tao Te Ching,* the Bhagavad-Gita, and the Koran, will provide a lifetime's worth of inspirational and strengthening passages. Favorite excerpts from poetry or music can be equally inspiring. If a particular phrase has remained with you for some time, chances are that it has touched some deep chord in you and may well be what you need to stimulate many positive associations and inner responses that are attempting to surface in your psyche.

Concentrate on a Single Image

Various types of single images can also be used to enter into deep relaxation and instill security and strength. The person who uses this type of meditation should "see" in his or her mind's eye the image in as much detail as possible. One should also "feel" the qualities associated with such images. Try to hold on to these feelings for as long as you can before you emerge from the meditation. Some of the images used to instill a sense of peace, strength, and longevity are a mountain, which is the picture of stillness, tranquillity, and strength; a pool of water, which can represent stillness, but also embraciveness; the ocean—the picture of primal power, the primordial mother of all life on the planet, which combines strength with serenity, patience, and longevity; a tree, with its peaceful, yet relentless growth and beauty; the grace and buoyancy of a single white cloud. Allow the positive associations of these and other images you may create intuitively to well up inside you; allow these feelings to fill your being with all the positive emotions and strength that they inspire.

Focus on Your Breath

This is an ancient spiritual practice that religious traditions of both East and West have encouraged for centuries. Once you have achieved a relaxed state, begin to concentrate on inhaling and exhaling your breath; see all the good, supportive, and strengthening energy of life travel into your body and fill up your lungs. Watch all undesirable emotions, sickness, and difficulties being discharged from your body and your life. Note the rhythmic quality of your breath — the expansion (inhalation) and contraction (exhalation) that take place in your body, as well as in all of life. With every breath, you align yourself more with the primal movements of the universe, the very basic expansion and contraction that take place on the grand scale, that of the cosmos itself, as well as on the microscopic level, where the movements of subatomic particles are governed by this alternating rhythm.

There are as many types of meditation as there are spiritual and religious practices. You may think of many other meditative devices that haven't been mentioned. The point is to achieve a deep state of relaxation while fostering the increase of positive emotions within you. (As noted in Chapter 5, vigorous exercise is an excellent way to relax as well.) These and the guided imagery techniques that follow can be done at any time of the day or night; all you need is a few minutes alone and a fairly comfortable chair to sit in. The rest is up to you and your ability to concentrate, which will improve dramatically as you become more adept at these practices.

After you have mastered these simple techniques you may want to move on to the four more complex and perhaps more rewarding meditations, which can be very powerful and strengthening. Some readers may find the guided imagery exercises a little difficult to master at first; they require more concentration and a certain amount of memorization. You can solve both of these problems, however, by recording the guided imagery routines on a cassette tape and simply listening to them, instead of trying to lead yourself through the exercises by memory. This can help you do the positive imaging routines until you feel ready to do them on your own. Of course, the short meditative exercises are a good way to work up to the more demanding techniques.

The four guided imagery exercises are the Relaxation Exercise, which can help you attain a deep state of relaxation and stimulates a wide array of positive associations and feelings; the Light Meditation, for those who are ill or lacking in vitality and would like to use positive imaging to help improve their condition; and two variations of a Spiritual Guide Meditation, which are designed to provide comfort, creative inspiration, and reconciliation.

Guided Imagery Exercise No. 1
The Relaxation Exercise

- Go to a softly lighted room and sit in a straight-backed comfortable chair. Take off your shoes and sit back.
- Take note of your breathing. Slow down your breathing so that your breath is drawn deep into your stomach and then release it in a very gradual and relaxed manner. Continue to breathe deeply and slowly.
- Focus your attention on the muscles in your face and concentrate on relaxing them. Feel your tension melt away. Feel the weight of your facial muscles as they become more relaxed.

- Turn your attention to the muscles of your neck and shoulders. Let your neck and shoulders relax and feel their weight. Feel the tension fall away from your neck and shoulders like great ice floes giving way under a warm sun.
- Let your arms rest comfortably, either in your lap or on the arms of the chair. Feel the energy and tension drain from them.
- Focus your attention on your stomach and chest. Your breathing should be slow, calm, and deep. Relax your stomach and chest and picture the tension falling away from your body.
- Concentrate your attention on your legs and feet. Once again, physically feel the tension dissipate, as if it were draining down your legs and out the bottoms of your feet.
- Feel warm, relaxed, and well.
- Now, picture a natural setting that holds particular beauty and peace for you. Is it an ocean or a forest? Are there rock formations or jetties on the beach, or a river in the forest? Fill in the details with your mind. See as clear and precise a picture as you can invent or remember. Listen to the sounds that are present in this place; feel the sun and gentle wind against your skin. Feel the peace and joy that this place creates in you. Notice any and all positive associations you may have here, and allow such feelings to well up within you.
- Concentrate on this image as long as you wish, continuing to feel the positive associations and emotions, and then gradually come out of the meditation.

Note: The setting can be different with each meditation; the only criterion is that you have positive associations and feelings about the place you allow your mind to go to while you are meditating. If you limit the number of settings you use, you come to know each place in greater detail, and you participate in the meditation to a greater extent than if the images are shallow or vague. Try as much as you can to involve your senses in your imaginary place.

Guided Imagery Exercise No. 2
The Light Meditation

■ Perform the Relaxation Exercise.
■ Imagine a small spark of light emanating from the cells of your heart.
■ Notice that this light is tiny but powerful.
■ Watch the spark of light gradually become larger, until it fills your entire chest area, then spreads to every part of your body, emanating from your every pore.
■ Imagine now that the cells of your body are radiant with light. This light is all-powerful and has an entirely energizing and transforming effect on your being, filling you with joy, love, and limitless energy. Hold this state for as long as you can or until you feel ready to let it go.

If you are in poor health, follow the steps below:

■ Notice that every cell within you which is ill cannot absorb the light; these cells are therefore dark and weak.
■ Picture your white blood cells, which are clothed in light, bearing down on the dark, weak, diseased cells. The light cells are infinitely more powerful, numerous, and organized than the dark cells.
■ Picture the light cells routing the diseased cells and forcing them into your digestive tract, where they will be eliminated from your body.
■ Picture a large but distinct source of light just above you. This source of light is infinitely radiant and has limitless power.
■ Imagine this source of light sending energy into your body, making you all the more radiant and filled with vitality.

■ Bathe in the warmth of this energy. It is love.
■ Continue the meditation until you feel ready to emerge from it.

The third guided imagery exercise is taken in part from the works of Dr. Raymond Moody, author of *Life After Life,* and Dr. Michael Sabom, a cardiologist and author of *Recollections of Death.* Moody stimulated enormous interest and controversy when he reported the experiences people had recalled during the period known as clinical death. (*Clinical death* is a term used to describe a state in which no external life signs, such as consciousness, heartbeat, respiration, and reflexes, are present.) Moody interviewed one hundred fifty people who had experienced clinical death, and he found that many of these people had remarkable and often similar memories of what they believed had happened to them during their periods of unconsciousness. These recollections included the separation of their consciousness from their bodies; a sense of enormous peace, freedom, and loss of pain; the ability to observe themselves and their surroundings from well above their own bodies while doctors and nurses attempted to resuscitate them; and, in the case of some, the sense of entering into a transcendent environment of extraordinary beauty, where they encountered relatives, friends, and a "being of light," whom many referred to as an angel, Christ, or simply God.

Sabom, who was highly skeptical of Moody's findings and methodology, was later persuaded to conduct a similar scientific study of his own. From 1976 to 1981 he interviewed more than one hundred people who had experienced clinical death and tested, whenever possible, the accuracy of their statements. For example, Sabom discovered that many of those who had near-death experiences could describe in remarkable detail the cardiopulmonary resuscitation (CPR) technique and the medical equipment used on them during clinical death. Many of these people explained that they had witnessed the medical procedures from a vantage point other than their bodies—from the door of the emergency room or from above their bodies, for example. Those who claimed to witness the procedure from the latter position gave remarkably accurate, virtually error-free answers. They were laypersons who had no prior knowledge of the medical procedures they underwent, and therefore could not be expected to give such detailed answers without having witnessed the procedure.

Sabom compared the accuracy of these descriptions to those of a control group of twenty-five patients who had undergone CPR, but who had not had the near-death experience. Nearly all of those in the control group made substantial errors in recounting what went on during CPR.

Like Moody, Sabom discovered that some of those who had near-death experiences also encountered a "spirit" or "presence," whom they often referred to as Christ, God, or an angel. Moody had reported that this transcendent figure reviewed the person's life in an atmosphere of enormous love and understanding. A few of the people in Sabom's study also reported undergoing some type of life review in which their lives flashed before them. Both Sabom and Moody found that many of those who had near-death experiences underwent dramatic changes in their anxiety and fear of death and experienced spiritual and religious conversion as a result. They believed that death was actually a pleasant and rewarding experience, and that life had a purpose. They also maintained that their experiences had taught them that God is present in their lives, providing support and guidance. Interested readers may want to consult the works cited for further details. Our purpose here is not to support or refute their findings or conclusions, but only to explain the source of the "transcendent figure," which is the focus of the next exercise.

The following meditation attempts to bring us into contact with a transcendent or spiritual guide. Jung maintained that each of us has a higher center within us, which he called the self. This self is continually guiding us toward resolution of conflicts and providing us with courage and a sense of well-being. Simonton, whom we mentioned earlier as a pioneer in the use of guided imagery in the treatment of cancer, has had success in using this "inner guide" as the principal subject of meditations designed to give people a sense of personal strength and support, both of which help to stimulate the will to live and the immune response. The meditation that follows can also be a great source of comfort and encouragement for those who face difficulties. People who adopt it will be surprised at the creative and inspirational responses they get from the transcendent figure or inner guide.

We recommend that you use either of the two images — the transcendent figure encountered in the near-death experiences, or Jung's inner guide — in the following meditations.

Guided Imagery Exercise No. 3
Spiritual Guide Meditation

- Perform the Relaxation Exercise.
- Imagine yourself alone in your peaceful setting, imbued with light.
- Feel the light fill your heart and entire being with love, energy, and comfort.
- In the distance you perceive a figure approaching; the figure is yours to choose — for example, it could be a man, a woman, or simply an orb of light. It, too, is resplendent in light, energy, and love. It approaches to help you.
- As the figure comes closer, you feel overcome with love for this being. You feel increasingly peaceful, relaxed, and filled with joy.
- You are aware of this transcendent figure's limitless wisdom. The being has all the qualities of Jesus, Buddha, Gandhi, or any other highly evolved being whom you admire.

- This figure is available for you to consult on any matter of importance to you.
- Present your problems and anxieties. When you are finished, imagine all your negative feelings about the difficulty leaving you, like dark clouds being released from your being, which evaporate and are gone.
- Listen carefully to the advice you receive from your spiritual guide. Gradually, you will come to understand the steps you must take to correct the situation that disturbs you.
- Spend as much time as you feel necessary with this being, then slowly emerge from the meditation.

Only saints can avoid conflict. Most of us are at one time or other filled with anger, resentment, and even hatred at the mere thought of some people. The following meditation can be helpful in letting go of these negative emotions.

Guided Imagery Exercise No. 4
Resolution of Conflict

- Perform the Relaxation Exercise and imagine yourself in your natural setting. (This meditation can include the presence of the transcendent figure, or you may choose to leave out the spiritual guide. It is purely up to you.)
- Imagine that the person with whom you are in conflict is present with you.
- Recognize that both of you have experienced much pain in life, which has made your past relationship difficult.
- Imagine a beam of light coming out of you, filling the other person with love and light. Feel your love for this person growing, making him or her stronger and more peaceful.
- Picture all your negative feelings toward this person emerging from you like dark clouds, which instantly dissipate and vanish.
- Picture yourself giving this person love and freedom.
- Imagine that both of you are happy and free.

- See the beam of light between you gradually fade, while the good feelings within both of you remain.
- Picture the person fading entirely from view.
- Feel yourself being filled with light, energy, and love, which is healing and supportive. (If you have chosen to include the spiritual guide in the meditation, listen to the advice this being gives you.)
- Focus on all the positive feelings inside you, and hold them for the rest of the meditation.
- Gradually emerge from your meditation, renewed.

As Jung and other professional counselors have found, such meditations release a barrage of images, symbols, and emotions. They will open doors for you that will prove to be rewarding and illuminating, but they may at times be unsettling and painful. For this reason, we caution you to proceed slowly and seek the advice of a trained counselor should issues emerge with which you feel unable to deal. In addition, do not hesitate to make changes in the routines to make them more rewarding, or better able to address the specific problems with which you are working.

Do not be discouraged if the guided images just don't appear to you at all. If you can master the relaxation exercise you will have accomplished a great deal. As with the diet and the physical exercises, every step you take will improve your health and well-being. The beauty of this program is that you don't have to master it to benefit from it. Remember, every step you *do* take makes it easier for you to move on to the next one when you are ready for it.

Chapter 8

A Program for Good Health

*H*OW CAN WE eat good food, exercise, and meditate all in the same day, and still have time to accomplish anything else? There is no one answer for everyone; you can arrive at the most appropriate regimen for your own lifestyle only by experimenting and moving at your own speed. At the same time, it is helpful to have a clear goal in mind, and for this reason we have included a seven-day schedule with a meal plan and suggestions for appropriate times for exercise and meditation. You do not have to follow this schedule strictly to benefit by it. You may repeat the program as often as you like or vary it to suit your own tastes, choosing from the lists of food in Chapter 3. Every time you exercise, every minute you meditate, every healthful meal you eat is a positive step that will benefit your health and peace of mind. Try each of the methods and ideas presented below and discover whether you are comfortable with them or how you might change them to suit your own needs. Allow twenty-one days to incorporate into your life as many of these ideas as you can. In three weeks you'll notice a surprising difference in your body and soul.

Chapter 10 contains recipes for all of the foods specified in the program, as well as for more exotic dishes that you'll want to try. Most of the foods prescribed in the program are basic and easy to prepare. Do not restrict yourself to the meal plans listed below; as much as possible, vary your cooking methods and experiment with the recipes. Should you crave a particular food that is not included in the diet, it's better to eat it and satisfy the craving rather than deny yourself and become so frustrated and preoccupied with your need that you jeopardize the whole program. However, we advise that you eat smaller portions of foods outside the diet, and that you eat them less frequently than you ordinarily would. Try to reduce, as much as possible, all foods that are high in fat, cholesterol, refined grains, sugar, and salt.

The more adept you become at preparing natural foods, the less time they will require and the more delicious your meals will be. Some short cuts follow.

- When you cook your dinner grain, prepare enough for at least two additional meals. If you cook brown rice for dinner one night, make enough for either breakfast or lunch the following day. (Reheat the breakfast grain with a little water to make it moister and easier to digest.)
- If you haven't time to prepare it, lunch the next day can be made up entirely of leftovers from the previous night's meal.
- Supper the following evening can also consist of the rice or other grain you cooked the night before. All you have to do is reheat your grain and steam or boil vegetables for a complete meal. (Steaming or boiling most vegetables requires 10 minutes or less.)
- Unlike boiling, which usually requires you to stand over the pot to protect the food from burning, pressure-cooking requires little or no attention once the food has come to pressure. Brown rice requires about 45 minutes to 1 hour of preparation time, while some beans take between 1 and 2 hours to cook; by using a pressure cooker you can allow

your grain or beans to cook while you are engaged in another activity.

- Take time during the weekend to cook foods that require longer preparation, then refrigerate them for use during the week. Refrigerated beans or seaweeds, for example, last for several days before they turn sour.
- Such condiments as roasted sesame seeds and dressings can also be prepared on the weekend and used throughout the week.
- To save time and still enjoy a delicious bean food, try tofu and tempeh. Both are rich in protein, vitamins, minerals, and carbohydrate. Tofu can be eaten raw in a variety of ways, and it is delicious in a sandwich with whole-grain bread and bean sprouts. (Tofu and the sprouts can be purchased in most supermarkets.) Tofu and tempeh are rich and satisfying foods that can be steamed, boiled, or broiled in 10 minutes.
- Some of the better natural food companies offer premade whole-grain mixes for such foods as tabbouleh (or tabouli, a Middle Eastern whole-wheat dish made with vegetables and spices), whole-wheat pancakes, grainburgers, and desserts. In addition, many desserts and snacks can be purchased ready-made in natural food and health food stores. While all these foods are essentially nothing more than natural fast foods, they are still healthier for you than standard fast-food fare. They also offer tasty and pleasant diversions from your routine.

Once you get into the habit of cooking natural foods, you'll find they require only slightly more time to prepare than your present diet, and they are far more rewarding.

You should take at least one brisk ten-minute walk per day and perform ten minutes of calisthenics or Do-In exercises, alternating from day to day. In addition, we urge you to seek out exercise wherever you may find it. Take stairs instead of elevators whenever possible; walk to the store and places where you do other errands. Park your car a distance from your destination. Join a spa, health club, or community center.

There are three good times a day—morning, noon, and evening—to meditate. You may find that only one of these times is appropriate for you, or that you can employ all three periods. These meditations can last for only five minutes and as long as half an hour. If you can find a quiet place and take five minutes at lunchtime, you may want to do the Relaxation Exercise. The effectiveness of the meditation depends more on your ability to focus, or concentrate, than it does on the amount of time you can devote to it. Your ability to concentrate will improve dramatically with regular use of these meditations, and five minutes during your lunch break is all you need to increase your peace of mind and equanimity during the workday.

All these activities—good diet, exercise, and meditation or prayer—will improve your health, vitality, and outlook. In short, they are the first steps toward a happier and healthier way of life.

The seven-day program follows.

Monday

The total amount of time required to prepare and eat breakfast, exercise, shower and dress, and meditate is approximately 2 hours, at most. You can shorten this period considerably if your breakfast grain needs only to be reheated. All the breakfast grains we recommend, like rolled oats and bulgur wheat, require 20 minutes or less to prepare. If you exercise for 10 minutes and meditate for 10 to 20 minutes, you have 1 hour and 10 minutes (minimum) to shower, dress, and eat. Here is a rough schedule.

Monday Morning

1. Exercise: 10 minutes of calisthenics or Do-In, as described in Chapter 4. (You can alternate calisthenics with Do-In every other day.)
2. Shower and dress: approximately 30 minutes
3. Meditation: Mornings afford an excellent time to do the Relaxation Exercise followed by the Light Meditation; however, if you use one of the shorter meditations, perform the meditation of your choice; meditate for 10 to 20 minutes.
4. *Menu:*
   Scrambled Tofu (see recipe under Beans in Chapter 10; takes about 10 minutes)
   Whole-grain toast with unsweetened jam or apple butter
   Kukicha (bancha) tea or grain coffee (may be sweetened with barley malt or yinnie syrup)
   Total preparation time: 20 minutes

Monday Noon

1. *Menu:*
   Bulgur wheat (cook it the night before; optional)
   Steamed broccoli and raw carrots or celery stalks
   Apple or some other fresh fruit
   Beverage (choose from the list of beverages in Chapter 3)
2. Walk: 10 minutes (optional, depending on the length of time you have for lunch)
3. Relaxation Exercise or meditation of your choice: 5 minutes (optional, depending on time)

Monday Evening

1. *Menu:*
   Pressure-Cooked or Boiled Brown Rice with Sesame Seed Condiment (can be cooked the night before; requires approximately 1 hour)

Sautéed greens and onions (greens can be kale, collard, mustard, cabbage, or others listed in Chapter 3; takes 10 minutes)

Baked Squash (acorn, butternut, or summer; can be cooked the night before and reheated; requires 1 hour)

Dried fruit cooked in apple juice, to make a sweet compote (10 to 15 minutes)

Total preparation time: 1½ hours maximum, from scratch

2. Evening walk
3. Evening meditation: Relaxation Exercise and Spiritual Guide Meditation or meditation of your choice (15 to 20 minutes)

Tuesday

Tuesday Morning

1. Do-In or calisthenics: 10 minutes
2. Shower and dress
3. Relaxation Exercise and Light Meditation or meditation of your choice
4. *Menu:*
   Rolled oats and raisins (requires 20 minutes, maximum)
   Whole-grain toast with unsweetened jam or apple butter
   Beverage

Tuesday Noon

1. *Menu:*
   Brown Rice with Sesame Seed Condiment (left over from Monday night's dinner)
   Sautéed greens (from Monday night's dinner)
   Salad with oil and vinegar or any dressing made from a recipe under Condiments and Dressings in Chapter 10
   Beverage
   Fresh fruit dessert

2. 10-minute walk (optional)
3. Relaxation Exercise or the meditation of your choice
   (optional; 5 minutes)

Tuesday Evening

1. *Menu:*
   Udon or other whole-wheat noodles with scallions (takes
     30 minutes to prepare)
   Steamed watercress, turnips, and Brussels sprouts (re-
     quires 15 minutes, including time to cut turnips)
   Fried Tempeh (cut into small chunks; 15 minutes)
   Coffee Gelatin Dessert (see recipe under Fruits and
     Desserts in Chapter 10; requires 20 minutes to prepare)
   Beverage
   Total preparation time: 45 minutes to 1 hour
2. Evening walk
3. Evening meditation: Relaxation Exercise and Spiritual
   Guide Meditation or meditation of your choice
   Note: While you are meditating, you can pressure-cook
   the grain for Wednesday night's dinner.

Wednesday

Wednesday Morning

1. Calisthenics or Do-In: 10 minutes
2. Shower and dress
3. Relaxation Exercise and Light Meditation or meditation
   of your choice
4. *Menu:*
   Bulgur and oatmeal (boiled together; requires 20
     minutes)
   Beverage

Wednesday Noon

1. *Menu:*
   Udon noodles with scallions (from Tuesday night's dinner)
   Steamed greens (from Tuesday night's dinner)
   Beverage
   Fresh fruit
2. 10-minute walk (optional)
3. Relaxation Exercise (optional) or meditation of your choice (5 minutes)

Wednesday Evening

1. *Menu:*
   Millet with Cauliflower, pressure-cooked or boiled together (see recipe under Whole Grains in Chapter 10; requires 45 to 60 minutes)
   Steamed greens and carrots (20 minutes)
   Baked sweet potato (requires 1 to 1½ hours)
   Fruit Gelatin Kanten (see recipe under Fruits and Desserts in Chapter 10; requires 20 minutes)
   Beverage
   Total preparation time: 1 hour 20 minutes
2. Evening walk
3. Evening meditation: Relaxation Exercise and Spiritual Guide Meditation or meditation of your choice.
4. Prepare grain for following couple of days (optional)

Thursday

Thursday Morning

1. Do-In or calisthenics
2. Shower and dress

3. Relaxation Exercise and Light Meditation or meditation of your choice
4. *Menu:*
    Whole-grain muffin with natural spread
    Beverage

Thursday Noon

1. *Menu:*
    Tofu sandwich on whole-grain bread with sprouts or lettuce, or leftover grain
    Steamed greens and raw celery stalks
    Fresh fruit
    Beverage
2. 10-minute walk (optional)
3. Relaxation Exercise or meditation of your choice

Thursday Evening

1. *Menu:*
    Pressure-Cooked or Boiled Brown Rice with Sesame Seed Condiment
    Steamed broccoli (10 minutes)
    Sautéed onions (requires 10 minutes to cut and sauté)
    Miso Soup with carrots, scallions, and dulse or wakame seaweed (see recipe under Beans, Chapter 10; requires 10 minutes)
    Fruit Crisp (fruit boiled in apple juice and topped with granola; requires 15 to 20 minutes)
    Total preparation time, from scratch: 1½ hours maximum
2. Evening walk
3. Relaxation Exercise and Spiritual Guide Meditation or meditation of your choice
4. Prepare a bean or grain for Friday (optional)

Friday

Friday Morning

1. Calisthenics or Do-In
2. Shower and dress
3. Relaxation Exercise and Light Meditation or meditation of your choice
4. *Menu:*
   Soft rice (reheated with a little water) and small amount of yinnie rice syrup to sweeten it (if desired)
   Beverage

Friday Noon

1. *Menu:*
   Rice with sesame seeds (from Thursday night's dinner)
   Salad with dressing
   Raw carrot sticks
   Beverage
2. 10-minute walk (optional)
3. Relaxation Exercise or meditation of your choice (optional)

Friday Evening

1. *Menu:*
   Vegetable Soup (see recipe under Vegetables, Chapter 10; requires 20 minutes)
   Noodles in Broth (see recipe under Whole Grains, Chapter 10; requires 25 minutes)
   Boiled greens (broccoli, mustard, or collard greens; requires 10 minutes to boil greens and roast sesame seeds)
   Roasted nuts and dried fruit

Beverage
Total preparation time: 35 to 40 minutes
2. Evening walk
3. Relaxation Exercise and Spiritual Guide Meditation or
   meditation of your choice

Saturday

Saturday Morning

1. Do-In or calisthenics
2. Shower and dress
3. Relaxation Exercise and Light Meditation or meditation
   of your choice
4. *Menu:*
   Oatmeal with raisins (requires 20 minutes)
   Whole-grain toast or muffin with jam
   Beverage

Saturday Noon

1. *Menu:*
   Buckwheat Burgers (or use leftover grain from week; see
   recipe under Whole Grains, Chapter 10; requires 25
   minutes)
   Steamed or sautéed onions and mushrooms (takes 20
   minutes)
   Salad with dressing
   Fresh fruit
   Beverage
   Total preparation time: 30 minutes
2. Some type of recreation or exercise: walking, golf, tennis,
   etc.

3. Relaxation Exercise or meditation of your choice
4. Prepare grain, bean, or condiment for the week ahead (optional)

Saturday Evening

1. *Menu:*
   Broiled Fish (see recipe under Animal Foods, Chapter 10; requires 25 minutes)
   Cornmeal (see recipe under Whole Grains, Chapter 10)
   Baked squash (requires 1 hour)
   Apple Crisp with Whipped Tofu Cream (see recipes under Fruits and Desserts, Chapter 10; requires 20 minutes, including whipping tofu)
   Beverage
   Total preparation time: 1½ hours
2. Evening walk (optional)
3. Relaxation Exercise and Spiritual Guide Meditation or meditation of your choice

Sunday

Sunday Morning

1. Light Do-In (nothing strenuous)
2. Relaxation Exercise and Light Meditation or meditation of your choice
3. Shower and dress
4. *Menu:*
   Whole-grain pancakes (mixes are available in most natural food and health food stores) with real maple syrup or barley malt
   Beverage

Sunday Noon

1. *Menu:*
    Noodle Salad (see recipe under Whole Grains, Chapter 10) with Creamy Tofu Dressing (see recipe under Condiments and Dressings, Chapter 10; requires less than 30 minutes)
    Steamed mustard greens with sunflower seeds
    Pressure-cooked or boiled beans with stalk of kombu seaweed (see Chapter 3, bean section; requires about 1½ hours to make from scratch, depending on type of bean used; to cut down time, substitute broiled, boiled, or steamed tempeh or tofu, which requires less than 20 minutes; make enough for meals during the week)
2. Light recreation or walk
3. Relaxation Exercise or meditation of your choice

Sunday Evening

1. *Menu:*
    Pressure-cooked or boiled barley with sesame seeds (requires 1 hour)
    Steamed carrots and Brussels sprouts
    Boiled rutabaga, cut into thin slices (requires 30 minutes)
    Steamed collard greens
    Coffee Gelatin (see recipe under Fruits and Desserts, Chapter 10)
2. Evening walk (optional)
3. Relaxation Exercise and Spiritual Guide Meditation or meditation of your choice.

Hope, Faith, and Love

This book began with a message of hope—that we have the power to make our lives better. Each of us can eat a healthier diet, exercise more, and try to cultivate a positive attitude toward life. The suggestions made here work; they are tools for change, but you have to be willing to experiment with them and use them as you see fit.

My own first steps on this path of self-transformation also began with hope, and with what I originally considered a very strange Eastern philosophical system. Initially, that system baffled and frightened me. I did not want to change, but I was forced into it for survival. I never dreamed, in September 1978, that I was on the brink of a far more rewarding life than I'd ever known. All I knew then was that I was being confronted with ideas that were foreign to my many ingrained beliefs. In a very real sense, my old life had to die, and I had to be willing to take up a new one if I was going to live at all. As I look back on the fall of 1978, I do so with gratitude and awe, because I see the creative power of life moving in me, and a process that seems to be everywhere in nature—that of letting old ways die and giving oneself over to the new.

Of course, change always means venturing into the unknown, something that frightens nearly everyone. To be able to make the changes encouraged by this book, one has to make a leap of faith. For this reason, we have tried to give you an abundance of scientific evidence to support our points, my own experience, and that of traditional cultures thousands of years old. We also caution you to proceed slowly and to adopt the program at your own natural speed. But to do anything in life, one must risk the security of the past and venture into the unknown. For this we need faith.

But the greatest power of transformation is love. Love changes everything it touches because giving love involves giving creative energy—energy that fosters growth and adaptability in whatever it goes out to. By eating better, exercising more, and cultivating a positive attitude toward life and the world around us, we fill our own lives, and everything with which we come in contact, with creative energy. We are, in essence, saying that we love life. It is not surprising, therefore, that such practices result in better health. But ultimately, it is only in giving of ourselves, letting go of our resistance to change, and being open to the gifts waiting for us in the new, that we begin to experience the true reward of living.

As Saint Paul wrote, "And now abideth in faith, hope, love, these three; but the greatest of these is love."

Mane Nobiscum Domine

Part II

Chapter 9

Cooking for Life

*T*HE KEY to preparing delicious natural foods lies in simplicity—use fresh and wholesome ingredients and don't overcook or overseason them. Allow their natural flavors to come out by using the easy methods we've mentioned before—pressure-cooking, steaming, boiling, sautéing, baking, broiling, and frying—and seasoning with natural condiments. The more simply you prepare your food, the better it will taste, and the more healthful it will be. Most of the recipes that follow do not require a chef's culinary talents. If you are not very adept in the kitchen, and I certainly am in that company, stick to the basic preparations in the beginning and then become more daring as you master these dishes. Most of the foods in the meal plan in Chapter 8 are uncomplicated dishes, and you shouldn't have any trouble preparing them.

It is very important that you vary your cooking methods and the grains and vegetables you eat. Concentrate on getting a wide variety of the three vegetable groups: leafy greens, of which kale, collard, and mustard greens are especially important; round and ground, of which the squashes, broccoli, cabbage, onions, and Brussels sprouts should be regulars at your table; and roots, especially carrots, turnips, rutabaga, and daikon.

Use the Sesame Seed Condiment (see recipe under Condiments and Dressings, Chapter 10) to enhance the flavor of your food. If you don't feel up to grinding the sesame seeds by hand or in a blender, simply follow the instructions for roasting them and sprinkle them over your grains. The seeds add a nutty and delicious taste to grains and combine with the grain to provide all the essential amino acids.

We also offer a few tips for good health that have more to do with the act of eating than with the food itself. First, try to eat when you are relaxed; eating while in an agitated state or standing makes it difficult for you to digest your food and prevents you from fully enjoying your meal. Relaxation is easily accomplished by taking a few deep breaths before you start to eat and allowing your breathing to become slow, deep, and steady. Try to chew your food as many as thirty-five times per mouthful, or as near that number as you can. The longer you chew, the more the natural flavors of the food will emerge, helping you to enjoy your food all the more. Perhaps more important is the fact that chewing is the first step in your body's digestion process. By chewing, you not only break the food down into digestible particles, but you also release digestive enzymes from your salivary glands that make the work of your stomach and intestines easier and more efficient. Try to avoid eating for at least three hours before you go to sleep, to allow your body time to digest your food before you retire. If you go to bed with a full stomach, your body will have to work to digest your food during the night, keeping you from deep and restful sleep. You will inevitably wake up the next morning feeling tired and irritable — not a great way to start the day.

You will find below a shopping list to assist you in obtaining the foods you need to begin the program. You may find this helpful, particularly if you have never shopped in a natural food or health food store before. All the foods listed below can be purchased in a good natural food store, and most of them, including some of the whole grains, virtually all of the vegetables, some beans, fruit, and snack items, fish and chicken, many beverages, and some of the foods needed to make condiments, are also available in your local supermarket.

You do not have to purchase all of the foods, especially if you plan to start off slowly on the Transition Diet. Also, the quantities you need will vary, depending on the size of your family and how fully you adopt the program. Wherever possible, we have provided information on the number of servings you can expect to get from a particular quantity of food.

A short list of kitchen supplies that you'll need to get started follows the shopping list. Except for a few items, you probably already own most of them, since they are standard in most kitchens, no matter what diet you prepare there.

A Shopping List
1. Whole Grains

Buy at least 1 pound of any or all of the grains listed below; generally speaking, 2 cups of grain provide 4 servings.

Brown rice
Bulgur wheat
Buckwheat (Kasha)
Barley
Millet
Oats
Cornmeal

Buy 2 packages of any of the following kinds of noodles. Note: Some noodles are sold in bulk in natural food stores; 1 pound of noodles provides at least 4 servings.

Whole-wheat noodles, any size or shape.
Whole-wheat udon; 1 8-ounce package contains enough for 3 to 4 servings.

Buckwheat noodles, or soba; 1 8-ounce package provides 3 to 4 servings.

1 or 2 loaves of any whole-grain bread.

2. Vegetables

Buy at least 1 pound of any or all of these fresh vegetables:

Collard greens
Kale
Mustard greens
Broccoli
Squash: butternut, acorn, yellow, or zucchini
Cabbage
Onions
Brussels sprouts
Carrots
Turnips
Rutabagas
Scallions (1 bunch will do)
Chives (1 bunch)
Parsley (1 bunch)
Daikon radish (Unlike all the other vegetables mentioned, daikon is rarely available in supermarkets and usually must be purchased in a natural food store. Your local grocer, if asked, may be able to stock it for you and other customers.)

3. Beans

Buy at least 1 pound of any or all of the following beans; 2 cups of beans provide approximately 4 servings.

Azuki beans
Chickpeas
Lentils

Split peas
Tofu; 1 package provides 2 to 3 servings.
Tempeh; 1 package provides 4 small servings.

4. Seaweed

Buy 1 package of any or all of the following seaweeds:

Arame
Hijiki
Nori
Wakame
Kombu (comes in stalks)

5. Animal Foods

Buy any of the following fish; determine the amount by the number people you are feeding; 1 pound of fish usually provides 3 to 4 small portions.

Sole
Halibut
Haddock
Flounder
Cod
Snapper
Tuna packed in spring water (without salt, if possible)
Chicken, preferably precut white meat

6. Condiments and Dressings

Purchase any or all of the following:

Sesame seeds; 1 pound provides enough seeds for several
  weeks' worth of condiments.
Small dried fish, such as chirimen iriko and dried sardines
Apple and rice vinegars

Tofu
Sesame, safflower, corn, and olive oils
Natural shoyu, or soy sauce
Natural tamari
Low-sodium miso
Small amounts of chives, parsley, garlic, and ginger root

7. and 8. Snacks, Fruits, and Desserts

Fresh fruit, including lemons and limes
Dried fruit, including raisins, apples, peaches, apricots,
  pears, and others
Fruit juices
Sunflower, pumpkin, and sesame seeds
1 jar yinnie syrup
1 jar barley malt syrup
1 jar apple butter or other fruit spread
1 jar real maple syrup (unsweetened and unadulterated)
Puffed grain, including puffed wheat, corn, and rice
Rice cakes
Popcorn (sold by the pound in natural food stores)
Any natural candies, of which there are a variety that do not
  include refined sugar
Unsweetened applesauce, made without artificial
  ingredients
Raw vegetables, including carrots, celery, and lettuce
1 pound whole-wheat pastry flour
1 pound whole-wheat flour

9. Beverages

Purchase any or all of the following drinks:

Grain coffee substitute
Noncaffeinated tea, such as Kukicha (bancha) twig tea

Vegetable juices
Fruit juices
Spring water

Kitchen Equipment

The list of kitchen equipment represents the standard utensils used in natural food cooking. This does not mean, however, that you have to run out immediately and spend a fortune on them. As you become more adept at preparing this wholesome cuisine, you'll naturally expand your array of pots, pans, skillets, and other utensils. We do recommend that when you purchase a new pot, it be made of stainless steel, as opposed to aluminum or nonstick coated. Stainless steel provides the finest-quality cookware; it doesn't scratch or chip easily, as do both aluminum and nonstick-coated pots and pans. It is difficult to dent and lasts a lifetime. We recommend that you completely eliminate cooking in chemically coated pots and pans, since they can chip or scratch, leaving shavings of the chemical in your food.

A cast-iron skillet is a wonderful investment in good health and high-quality cookware. Cast-iron utensils have to be seasoned to keep them from flavoring your food with too much iron. To season your cast-iron pan, coat it with oil and fry an onion or other vegetable in it; when the vegetable is brown, throw it away and bake the pan in the oven at 250°F for a few hours.

List of Utensils

1 pressure cooker. A 5-quart pressure cooker is the most versatile; the pot, without its special lid, can be used for boiling. A pressure cooker with a screw-on lid, the type in

which the lid actually fits inside the pot (not around the top of the outside, as in most such pots), is extremely safe and virtually accident-free when used properly.

1 large stainless-steel pot for boiling and steaming

1 medium-sized cookie sheet for baking squash and desserts

1 medium-sized baking pan for baking beans and other foods

1 medium-sized pot for boiling and steaming small quantities of food

1 cast-iron skillet

1 heat spreader or diffuser, to keep the heat even under your pots and prevent the food from burning

1 colander—a perforated pot in which to wash grains and vegetables

3 wooden spoons of varying size to stir cooking food. Wooden spoons are preferable to steel or aluminum because they do not scratch the pots and are light and easy to use.

1 good vegetable knife. A must in any kitchen. A carbon-coated blade is about the best available; it resists chipping and keeps a fine edge longer. A sharpening stone is also a handy item for keeping a good edge on your knives.

1 vegetable brush. Wash, rather than peel, vegetables. Brushes made of natural ingredients are best.

1 wooden chopping block on which to cut vegetables and other foods. Wipe the board down with oil occasionally to keep it from cracking.

1 suribachi bowl (one with a serrated interior, excellent for grinding seeds and grain) and surikogi—a Japanese mortar and pestle—an ordinary mortar and pestle, or a blender. Any one of these can be used to grind sesame seeds and other foods into a fine grainy powder for condiments.

Natural fiber mats (the best are made from bamboo stalks) with which to cover food

1 vegetable grater

1 bamboo strainer to strain Kukicha (bancha) twig tea and other beverages

Large glass jars for storing supplies. Use the containers from apple juice and other foods. Glass jars keep grains, beans, and seeds dry and create a pleasing display of these colorful products. Keep your grains and seeds in a cool, dry place in your home to ensure that they remain unspoiled.

Chapter 10

The Recipes

*T*HIS CHAPTER CONTAINS more than fifty natural food recipes, which are organized into seven sections, following the order of the foods presented in Chapter 3. They represent a wide variety of dishes, and we do recommend that you eat widely, within the guidelines established in Chapters 2 and 3. Don't restrict yourself to just the dishes presented here; we encourage you to experiment with the menu plans outlined in Chapter 8 and the recipes. It takes some time to recognize that there is a world of variety waiting in natural food cuisine. Give yourself time to understand how to prepare these foods, and your palate time to adjust to the new flavors. Once you've mastered the basics, a lifetime of creative cooking awaits you.

Whole Grains
Pressure-Cooked Brown Rice

Pressure-cooking brings out the full delicious flavor of the grain and locks in all the important nutrients. Pressure-cooked rice, which has a stickier consistency than boiled rice, is wonderful for dinner.

> 2 cups brown rice (short, medium, or long grain)
> 3 cups water
> 1 small pinch salt
> 2 tablespoons roasted sesame seeds (optional)

Wash the rice in a pressure cooker several times, until the water runs clear. Drain. Add the water and salt, cover, and bring to full pressure over high heat. Slip a heat diffuser under the pot, reduce the heat to low, and simmer for 45 minutes. Turn off the heat, let pressure come down, and remove the rice. (Some of the rice at the bottom of the pot may have burned; be careful when removing rice that you do not mix the burned grain with the rest of the rice.) Add sesame seeds if desired.
   Serves 4 to 6

Variations

For a softer breakfast rice, use 2½ to 3 cups of water to 1 cup of rice and simmer for 1 hour. You can also reheat pressure-cooked rice with a little more water to make it softer.

   Use rice with millet, bulgur wheat, or vegetables like carrots, squash, or onions.

Boiled Brown Rice

Simmering, which produces fluffier rice than pressure-cooking, is recommended for hot days.

> 2 cups brown rice (short, medium, or long grain)
> 4 cups water
> 1 pinch salt

Wash the rice in a colander several times, until the water runs clear. Place all the ingredients in a pot and bring rapidly to a boil over high heat. Slip a heat diffuser under the pot, reduce the heat to medium or low, cover, and simmer for 45 minutes.

Turn off the heat and let stand covered for 5 minutes. Stir from the bottom to the top to mix the rice evenly. Serve with Sesame Seed Condiment (see recipe under Condiments and Dressings).

Serves 4 to 6

Variation

For a softer breakfast rice, use 4 cups of water to 1 cup of rice and simmer for 1½ hours. Serve with any of a variety of condiments

Breakfast Bulgur and Oatmeal

This recipe produces a sweet and sticky morning cereal.

> 4 cups water
> 1 cup bulgur
> 1 cup rolled oats
> ¼ cup raisins (optional)
> 1 pinch salt
> 1 pinch cinnamon

Bring the water to a boil, then add all the ingredients. Return to a boil, cover the pot, and slip a heat diffuser under the pot. Reduce the heat to medium and simmer for 20 to 30 minutes. Stir from the bottom to the top of the pot.

Serves 2 to 4

Dinner Bulgur

This recipe produces a fluffy dinner grain.

> 3 cups water
> 2 cups bulgur
> 1 pinch salt

Bring water to a boil in a pot, and add the bulgur and a few grains of salt. Cover, slip a heat diffuser under the pot, and simmer over low heat for 20 minutes. Garnish with sliced scallions or sprinkle with Sesame Seed Condiment (see recipe under Condiments and Dressings).

Serves 4 to 6

Buckwheat or Kasha

A hearty dish for cold days.

> 1 cup white buckwheat groats
> 2½ cups boiling water
> 1 pinch salt
> 1 onion, diced (optional)

Roast the buckwheat groats evenly in a frying pan for 4 to 5 minutes. (Roasting the grain brings out a nuttier flavor.) Place the roasted buckwheat in a pot and add the water, salt, and onion. Cover with a tight-fitting lid, slip a heat diffuser under the pot, reduce the heat to medium, and simmer for 30 minutes or until all the water has been absorbed. Stir from the bottom to the top. Serve with chopped raw scallions and sprinkle with Sesame Seed Condiment.

Serves 2 to 4

Buckwheat Burgers

> 3 cups cooked buckwheat groats (see recipe for Buckwheat)
> 1 cup minced onions
> ½ cup minced parsley
> ¼ cup grated mushrooms
> ½ pound tofu, mashed
> 1 clove garlic, minced (optional)
> 1 teaspoon natural soy sauce
> ¼ teaspoon basil (optional)
> 2 tablespoons sesame oil
> Pastry flour

Place all the ingredients, except the oil and flour, in a large bowl. Mix evenly with a wooden spoon. Add just enough pastry flour to hold the mixture together. If the mix gets too dry, add a little water. Form 1-inch-thick patties with wet hands. Heat the oil in a large skillet or frying pan. Fry the patties over medium-high heat on both sides until golden brown, approximately 8 to 10 minutes on each side. Shake the pan gently to prevent the patties from sticking. Reduce the heat if the patties get too dark. Makes 8 medium-sized patties. Serve on lettuce leaves with red onion rings and a dab of ketchup. (Ketchups made of all-natural ingredients and containing no sugar are available in most natural food and health food stores.)

Serves 4 to 6

Wheat Meat (Seitan)

Wheat meat is made from the gluten (protein) of wheat flour. It is very high in protein, carbohydrate, calcium, and B vitamins.

> 3 cups whole-wheat flour
> 3 cups unbleached white flour
> 3½ cups water (amount of water may vary, depending on type of flour and how it is milled)

Place the flours in a large bowl and mix well. Slowly pour in the water, stirring vigorously with a wooden spoon to form a soft, sticky dough. Knead the dough from the bottom to the top with one hand while slowly turning the bowl with the other. Rinse the hand used for kneading with cold water occasionally to prevent the dough from sticking to it. Kneading activates the gluten and makes the dough elastic. Do it for 8 minutes. Cover the dough with cold water and let soak for 30 minutes, minimum; dough may soak for up to 8 hours. Knead the dough again in the soaking water, adding more water to fill the bowl. Keep the dough in one piece by pushing from the outside toward the center. This kneading process extracts the bran and starch, and the water will become milky white. Store the starch water in the refrigerator and use it for stews, gravies, and puddings. Place the dough in a colander and continue kneading under cold running water until all the starch and bran are washed out. You will end up with a large, sticky ball (approximately 2 to 2½ cups' worth) of gluten. Cover it with water and refrigerate it until you are ready to use it in stews, with noodles, in soups, or by itself. Seitan can be stored for a week in the refrigerator.

You can cut the gluten, or seitan, in any shape or size you like and use it in any of the following recipes.

Flavored Wheat Meat or Seitan

Flavored wheat meat can be broiled, barbecued, and batter-fried and used in soups, salads, stews, casseroles, with sautéed vegetables, and in sandwiches. Combined with bread crumbs, onions, celery, and mushrooms, it makes an excellent stuffing for squash and peppers.

> 6 cups water
> 1 strip kombu
> ⅛ cup soy sauce
> 2 slices ginger (optional)
> 2 cloves garlic (optional)
> 2 cups raw wheat meat, cut into large pieces

Bring the water to a boil in a pot with the kombu, soy sauce, ginger, and garlic. Add the wheat meat, return to a boil, cover, and simmer over medium-low heat for 1 hour. Uncover and boil off the liquid over high heat. Store in the refrigerator.

Wheat Meat Cutlets with
Onion-Mushroom Gravy

Delicious served over rice, millet, noodles, or potatoes.

        2 tablespoons sesame oil
        2 cloves garlic, minced
        2 large onions, finely sliced
        2 cups sliced mushrooms
        7 cups water
        ⅛ cup soy sauce
        2 cups wheat meat, sliced into 10 cutlets
        ¼ teaspoon ground coriander
        1 dash nutmeg
        ½ cup wheat meat starch water

Heat the oil in a large skillet or frying pan and sauté the garlic, onions, and mushrooms, stirring constantly. Add the water and soy sauce and bring to a boil. Place the wheat meat cutlets in the water and return to a boil. Add the coriander and nutmeg, cover, and simmer over medium-low heat for 40 minutes. The wheat meat will expand during cooking. Pour the starch water evenly over the cutlets, stir gently, cover, and simmer over low heat for 10 minutes to make the gravy. If it's not thick enough, add a little more starch water.

Serves 5 to 8

Breakfast Cornmeal or Polenta

        3 cups water
        1 cup cornmeal (may be dry roasted for nuttier flavor),
            mixed with 1 cup cold water
        1 pinch salt

Bring the water to a boil in a pot. Whisk in the cornmeal mixture, add a few grains of salt, return to a boil, and stir continually to prevent lumping. Cover, slip a heat diffuser under the pot, and simmer over medium-low heat for 30 to 45 minutes. (Cooking time depends on how coarsely grain is ground.) Sprinkle with toasted sunflower seeds or Sesame Seed Condiment. For a sweet breakfast, add maple syrup, yinnie rice syrup, or barley malt.

Serves 4

Variation

Dessert Cornmeal Pudding: Substitute apple juice for water, add ¼ cup raisins or currants, and 1 teaspoon grated lemon rind. Delicious hot or cold.

Dinner Polenta Aspic with Vegetables

Great for lunch, dinner, picnics, and parties.

    1 red onion, minced
    1 medium carrot, cubed
    1 stalk celery, diced
    1 cup water
    1 clove garlic, minced (optional)
    1 pinch salt
    1 recipe Cornmeal or Polenta (see preceding recipe)

Wash and cut the vegetables. Place them in a saucepan and add seasoning. Cover with the water, and bring to a boil. Cover and simmer over medium-low heat for 5 minutes. Strain the vegetables (save the water for soup). Rinse a flat pan or baking dish in cold water. Arrange the cooked vegetables on the bottom of the pan and pour the hot cornmeal mixture over them. Cool for 1 hour or until the cornmeal sets. Cover the pan with a platter, turn it upside down, and shake gently back and forth until the polenta slips out. Cut into squares.

Serves 4 to 6

Pressure-Cooked Millet with Cauliflower

    1 cup millet
    ½ cauliflower
    2 tablespoons roasted sunflower seeds (optional)
    4 cups water
    2 pinches salt

Wash the millet in a strainer several times. Wash the cauliflower and cut it into flowerets. Place the cauliflower and sunflower seeds on the bottom of a pressure cooker, add the millet on top, and gently pour the water into one side of the pot to keep the layering intact. Add the salt and cover. Bring rapidly to full pressure over high heat, slip a heat diffuser under the pot, reduce the heat to medium-low, and simmer for 30 minutes. Bring down the pressure and stir from the bottom to the top of the pot. For a mashed-potato-like consistency, pass the food through a food mill. Garnish with chopped parsley or sliced scallions.
    Serves 4 to 6

Variation
Substitute 1 cup sweet squash (acorn, buttercup, or butternut) or 1 cup diced onion for the cauliflower.

Noodles in Broth

On hot summer days, chill this broth and serve it over cold noodles.

    1 8-ounce package wheat noodles (udon)
    6 cups water
    1 tablespoon soy sauce
    2 to 4 tablespoons bonito fish flakes (optional)
    ¼ teaspoon fresh ginger juice or grated ginger root
    (optional)
    3 scallions, thinly sliced

Add the noodles to boiling water and cook for 15 to 25 minutes or until soft. Do not cover. Strain the noodles by pouring the broth into another pot; hold a colander or strainer over the second pot to catch any noodles that come out with the broth. Rinse the noodles in the colander with cold water to prevent them from sticking. Then place the pot containing the broth on a burner and bring it to a boil, add the soy sauce, fish flakes, and ginger juice or root, and simmer over low heat for 5 minutes. Return the noodles to the broth and serve piping hot. Garnish with scallions.

Serves 2 to 4

Variation
Substitute buckwheat noodles (soba), or any other spaghetti-type noodle, for udon.

Noodle Salad

2 cups noodles (any variety)
½ cup carrots
½ cup peas
½ cup corn kernels

Dressing
½ pound tofu, raw
1 tablespoon sesame tahini (available in natural food stores; tahini, which is derived from sesame seeds, is similar to peanut butter.)
2 tablespoons light miso
1 tablespoon lemon juice
¼ cup water

¼ cup raw sliced scallions
1 tablespoon roasted sesame seeds

Boil the noodles, and drain the water. Wash the vegetables and dice the carrots. (In winter you may want to use frozen corn and peas.) Boil the vegetables for 2 minutes and drain the water. Cream the tofu, tahini, miso, lemon juice, and water in a suribachi or blender. Mix the tofu dressing with the cooked noodles and vegetables in a large bowl. Garnish with scallions and sesame seeds.

Serves 4 to 6

Leftover Grain Bread

No yeast, no baking powder, no oil required.

⅛ teaspoon salt
3 cups whole-wheat flour
3 cups leftover rice or other grain
1½ cups cold water
Flour for kneading

Place the salt, flour, and leftover grain in a bowl. Mix until all the grain is coated with flour. Gradually add the water, stirring constantly. Mix well and knead on a floured surface until the dough is elastic and has an even consistency. Fill two oiled bread pans three-quarters full, cover with a damp cloth, and let sit in a warm spot for 10 to 15 hours or until the dough has risen and smells slightly sour. Preheat the oven to 350°F, brush the tops of the dough with oil, and bake for 1 to 1½ hours. Tap slightly on the crusts. When the sound is hollow, the bread is done. Remove the loaves immediately and cool for 1 hour.

Yields 2 loaves

Variation

Substitute whole-wheat pastry flour and a small amount of cornmeal for whole-wheat flour to make a lighter bread.

Vegetables
Sautéed Leafy Greens

1 bunch leafy greens
2 to 3 tablespoons sesame oil
1 clove garlic, minced
½ cup sliced mushrooms
Few drops soy sauce
¼ teaspoon lemon juice
2 tablespoons ground roasted sesame or sunflower seeds

Wash the greens thoroughly. If you use large ones, cut them in half lengthwise along the side stem, stack them on top of each other, and cut again lengthwise. Turn them sideways and cut them into ½-inch pieces. Heat the oil in a frying pan and sauté the garlic until slightly brown. Add the mushrooms and stir for 2 minutes or until the mushrooms release their liquid. Add the greens and stir gently over high heat until they change color. Cover and simmer over medium-low heat for 2 minutes. Add the soy sauce and lemon juice, turn up the heat, and cook until most of the liquid has evaporated. Mix in the seeds and serve immediately.
Serves 4

Boiled Leafy Greens

1 bunch leafy greens
1 pinch salt
1 tablespoon ground roasted sesame seeds (optional)

Wash the greens and cut them into ½-inch pieces, as in the preceding recipe. Place them in a pot, add 1 inch of water, and bring to a boil. Add the salt, cover, and cook for 2 minutes. (Kale may be cooked longer — up to 5 minutes.) Sprinkle the greens with the sesame seeds.
Serves 4

Watercress with Tofu

2 bunches watercress
½ block (8 ounces) soft tofu, drained
1 teaspoon sesame oil
1 teaspoon soy sauce
Few drops brown rice vinegar (optional)

Wash the watercress and cut it into ½-inch pieces. Mash the tofu in a bowl with a fork. Heat the oil in a skillet or frying pan, add the mashed tofu and soy sauce, and stir over high heat until the liquid has almost evaporated. Add the watercress and gently mix with the tofu until the greens become limp — about 1 minute. Do not cover. Add a few drops of vinegar, stir, and serve immediately.

Serves 4

Variation

Use spinach instead of watercress.

Baked Squash

Good for fall and winter.

1 large acorn squash, cut in half
Corn oil for brushing

Wash and cut the squash. Remove the seeds. Place the squash on a cookie sheet, cut side down. Brush the skin with oil to prevent drying and bake in a preheated 350° to 375°F oven for 45 minutes or until soft. Test by pricking the ends of the squash with a toothpick.

Serves 4

Variation

Substitute butternut or any other squash for acorn.

Chinese-Style Vegetables

The thinner you cut these vegetables, the faster the cooking time, and the more delicate the flavor.

    3 tablespoons sesame oil
    ½ cup thin matchstick-sized pieces of carrot
    ½ cup thinly sliced celery
    ½ cup trimmed snow peas
    ½ cup thinly sliced mushrooms
    1 tablespoon soy sauce
    1 teaspoon arrowroot flour, dissolved in ¼ cup water
    1 bunch spinach, cut into bite-sized pieces
    1 cup bean sprouts, rinsed several times

Wash and cut the vegetables. Heat the oil in a wok or frying pan, and add the vegetables one at a time, starting with the carrots. Sauté the carrots over high heat for 1 minute or until the color changes. Remove the carrots with a slotted spoon and set aside. Continue with the celery, snow peas, and mushrooms, then combine the sautéed vegetables. Add the soy sauce and arrowroot mixture. Gently mix in the spinach and bean sprouts. Turn off the heat and serve immediately.
  Serves 4

Variation
Add 1 cup cubed tofu or flavored cubed wheat meat.

Boiled Daikon

    1 medium-sized daikon radish, cut into 1-inch-thick
      rounds
    Water
    1 tablespoon ground roasted sesame seeds
    Parsley
    Few drops soy sauce

Wash and cut the daikon. If the top is fresh, use it in the recipe. Place the daikon in a pot and cover it with water. Bring to a boil, cover, and simmer over medium-low heat for 30 minutes. Sprinkle with the sesame seeds, garnish with parsley, and season with soy sauce.

Serves 4

Spring and Summer Boiled Salad

The vegetables for boiled salad turn out most delicious when they are boiled individually, rather than thrown in all at once. Vegetables can each be boiled 1 or 2 minutes before removing them and adding another one to the same water.

> 6 cups water
> Few drops tamari or soy sauce
> 1 cup finely sliced celery, cut diagonally
> 1 stalk broccoli, cut into small flowerets
> 1 carrot, cut into matchstick-sized pieces
> 1 cup finely sliced onions, cut lengthwise
> 1 cup finely sliced purple cabbage

Bring the water to a boil in a pot and add a few drops of tamari or soy sauce. Add the celery and boil for 1 to 2 minutes or until its color brightens. Vegetables should be slightly crisp but not raw. Remove the celery with a slotted spoon, place it in a strainer with a plate underneath to catch the excess water. Repeat the same process with the broccoli, carrot, onions, and cabbage. Mix all the vegetables together in a large bowl and toss gently with your favorite dressing.

Serves 6 to 8

Vegetable Stew

An excellent dish for cold days.

> 1 large carrot, cut into 1-inch rounds
> 2 onions, cut into quarters
> 1 large yam, cut into 1-inch chunks
> ¼ head white cabbage, cut into 2-inch-thick pieces
> 1 strip kombu seaweed, soaked and cut into 1-inch pieces
> 2 small slices ginger (optional)
> 1 tablespoon white miso, creamed in 3 tablespoons water
> 2 tablespoons kuzu, arrowroot, or unbleached white flour, creamed in ¼ cup water

Wash and cut the vegetables. Place the kombu and ginger on the bottom of a large pot. Arrange the vegetables on top of the kombu, add 2 inches of water, and bring to a boil. Cover and simmer over medium-low heat for 30 minutes. Combine the creamed miso with the kuzu, arrowroot, or flour mixture, pour over the vegetables, and shake the pot gently back and forth to distribute the thickener evenly. Do not stir, as that will break the vegetables. Simmer for 10 minutes. Garnish with scallions. Remove the ginger slices before serving.

Serves 2 to 4

Variation
Use Brussels sprouts, turnips, rutabagas, squash, cauliflower, carrots, and other hearty vegetables, but try to limit the dish to only four vegetables.

Vegetable Soup

1½ cups thinly sliced leeks
1½ cups cubed carrots
½ cup cubed daikon radish
1 strip kombu, soaked and cut into small strips
1 pinch salt
6 cups water
2 tablespoons soy sauce or white miso

Wash and cut the vegetables. Give special attention to the leeks, which tend to be very sandy. If the green parts of the leeks are fresh, use them in the soup. Place the kombu, carrots, and daikon in a saucepan. Add the salt and water and bring to a boil. Reduce the heat to medium-low and simmer for 15 minutes. Add the leeks and leek greens, return to a boil, and simmer for 8 minutes. Season with the soy sauce or miso and simmer for another 5 minutes. (If you use miso, cream it with soup broth and add to the soup.) All the vegetables should be a bright color. Garnish with parsley. Serve with croutons made of roasted or fried whole-grain bread.

Serves 4 to 6

Variation

Add cooked noodles, beans, soft grain, or dumplings.

Creamy Squash Soup

1 large butternut squash, cut into 1-inch-thick chunks
1 large yam, cut into 1-inch-thick chunks
6 cups water
1 pinch salt
1 bunch scallions, thinly sliced
1 tablespoon soy sauce (optional)
¼ teaspoon fresh ginger juice or ⅛ teaspoon ginger powder
Dash nutmeg (optional)

Wash and cut the vegetables. Remove the seeds from the squash. Place the squash and the yam in a pot, add the water and salt, and bring to a boil. Cover and simmer over medium-low heat for 30 minutes. Take out the vegetables with a slotted spoon and pass them through a food mill or fine mesh strainer. The peel will remain in a strainer. (If you use a blender to cream them, peel the vegetables prior to cooking.) Return the creamed vegetables to the pot and stir well. Add the scallions, soy sauce, ginger, and nutmeg, bring to a boil, and simmer for 5 minutes. Sprinkle with roasted sunflower seeds and garnish with parsley.

Serves 4

Beans

Azuki Beans with Squash and Kombu

Kombu seaweed adds minerals that make beans easy to digest.

- 2 cups azuki beans
- 7 cups water
- 4 cups sweet squash (acorn, butternut, or any variety)
- 2 strips kombu seaweed, soaked in water
- 1 pinch salt or 1 teaspoon soy sauce

Pick over the dry beans, wash them several times, and drain. Soak the beans for 6 to 8 hours in 7 cups of water. Wash the squash and, if the skins are waxed, peel. Remove the seeds from the squash and cut it into 1-inch cubes. Cut the kombu into bite-sized pieces. Drain the beans, reserving the water in which they were soaked. Place the kombu, then the squash and beans in the bottom of a heavy pot. Gently pour the soaking water into one side of the pot, to keep the layering intact. Bring to a gentle boil, cover, and simmer over medium-low heat for 1 hour or until the beans are soft. Add the salt or soy sauce toward the end of the cooking time and simmer 10

minutes more. If too much liquid remains, turn up the heat and boil off the water. Garnish with freshly sliced scallions.
Serves 6

Pressure-Cooked Chickpea Soup

Pressure-cooking is the best method for preparing chickpeas because they are the hardest beans and require the longest cooking time.

> 2 cups chickpeas
> 8 cups water
> 1 strip kombu seaweed, soaked in water
> 1 bay leaf (optional)
> 1 cup diced onions
> 1 cup cubed carrots
> 1 cup diced celery
> 1 cup small cauliflower flowerets
> 1 clove garlic, minced (optional)
> 1 pinch salt or 1 teaspoon shoyu or 1 rounded tea-
>   spoon light miso, creamed in ¼ cup chickpea broth

Pick over the dry beans, wash several times, and drain. Soak the beans for 10 to 12 hours in 8 cups of water. Place the beans, soaking water, kombu, and bay leaf in a pressure cooker and bring to a boil, without the lid fastened. Skim off the foam. Cover the pressure cooker, place over high heat, and bring to full pressure. Reduce the heat to medium-low and simmer for 1½ hours. While the beans are cooking, wash and cut the vegetables. Place them in a pot with 3 inches of water, bring to a boil, and simmer for 5 minutes. Add the vegetables, garlic, and salt to the cooked beans and simmer together for 30 minutes. If the soup is too thick, add more water. For a creamy soup, mash the beans in the pot with a wooden spoon or pestle. Garnish with parsley.
Serves 6 to 8

Kidney Bean Salad

This salad is good for warm-weather parties and picnics.

    2 cups kidney beans
    7 cups water
    1 bay leaf
    1 red onion, minced
    2 stalks celery, diced
    2 cups sweet corn kernels
    1 cup diced carrots
    1 cup chopped parsley
    ⅛ teaspoon salt

Marinade
    3 tablespoons olive or corn oil
    2 tablespoons sweet brown rice vinegar or apple cider
      vinegar
    1 clove garlic, minced
    1 tablespoon soy sauce
    ½ teaspoon basil (optional)
    ⅛ teaspoon salt (optional)

Pick over the dry beans, wash them several times, and drain. Soak the beans for 8 hours in 7 cups of water, or boil them for 5 minutes and soak for 2 hours. Place the beans, soaking water, and bay leaf in a heavy pot, bring to a boil, cover, and simmer over medium-low heat for 1 hour or until the beans are soft. Stir occasionally, being careful not to mash the beans, to prevent them from sticking to the bottom of the pot. While the beans are cooking, wash and cut the vegetables. When the beans are completely soft, add the vegetables (and salt) and simmer together for 5 minutes. Drain any excess liquid (save it for soup), and place the mixture in the refrigerator to chill. Prepare the marinade by combining all the ingredients. Mix gently with the chilled bean salad and let sit for at least 30 minutes. Garnish with fresh sliced scallions and serve on a bed of lettuce.

Serves 6

Variation
Use chickpeas, pinto beans, or navy beans.

Tofu

Tofu makes a tasty addition to soups, stews, casseroles, sandwiches, and sautéed vegetables. It is readily available in supermarkets and natural food and health food stores. When storing tofu in the refrigerator, cover it with water and change the water daily. It will keep fresh for approximately five days.

Fried Tofu

Tasty in sandwiches, as a side dish, over noodles, and as an addition to soups.

> 1 8-ounce block tofu, drained
> 1 tablespoon sesame oil
> ¼ cup water
> 1 teaspoon soy sauce

Cut the tofu in ½-inch-thick slices. Heat the oil in a frying pan and fry the tofu on both sides until golden brown. Mix the water with the soy sauce, pour over the tofu, and cook over high heat until all the liquid has evaporated.

Serves 2

Scrambled Tofu (Mock Scrambled Eggs)

Try this dish instead of eggs for breakfast. Turmeric gives it its yellow scrambled-egg appearance and delicious flavor.

    1 tablespoon sesame oil
    3 scallions, thinly sliced
    2 8-ounce blocks tofu, drained and mashed
    1/8 teaspoon turmeric
    1 teaspoon soy sauce

Heat the oil in a frying pan, add the sliced scallions, and sauté for 1 minute. Add the mashed tofu and turmeric, place over high heat, and cook, stirring, for 5 minutes. Add the soy sauce and cook off any excess water.

Serves 2 to 3

Baked Tofu and Macaroni

    1 teaspoon sesame oil
    1 onion, diced
    1 small butternut squash, peeled and cubed
    1/2 cup water
    1 8-ounce block tofu, drained
    1/4 cup tahini
    3 tablespoons kuzu or arrowroot, dissolved in 1/4 cup
      water
    1 tablespoon white miso
    1/2 teaspoon basil
    4 cups cooked elbow noodles

Heat the oil in a frying pan and sauté the onion for 2 minutes. Add the squash and the water and steam for 10 minutes or until the squash is soft. Place the remaining ingredients, except the noodles and basil, in a blender, and whip until creamy. Add the basil, combine the tofu mixture with the cooked noodles, and turn into an oiled casserole. Cover and bake in a 350°F preheated oven for 20 minutes. Uncover and allow the top to brown for about 10 minutes. Garnish with parsley.

Serves 4 to 6

Tofu and Sweet Corn

Sesame oil
2 cups sweet corn kernels
2 8-ounce blocks tofu, drained and cubed
¼ teaspoon soy sauce

Brush a skillet or frying pan lightly with sesame oil. Add the corn and sauté for 2 minutes. Layer the cubed tofu over the corn, cover, and simmer for 5 minutes. Season with soy sauce and mix together gently.

Serves 4 to 6

Variation

Add onions, green peas, or spinach to the tofu and corn.

Tempeh

Tempeh is a fermented soybean product that comes in a six-inch-square patty, perhaps one-half inch thick. It is high in protein, carbohydrates, B vitamins, and important bacteria that aid digestion; tempeh also contains vitamin B_{12}. It can be purchased in most natural food and many health food stores. Like tofu, tempeh can be fried, deep-fried, boiled, broiled, baked, and sautéed. It makes a wonderful addition to soups, stews, salads, noodles, and sandwiches.

Fried Tempeh Sandwich

½ block (4 ounces) tempeh
1 tablespoon corn oil
½ cup water
1 teaspoon soy sauce
2 slices toasted whole-grain bread
mustard (optional)
mayonnaise (optional; mayonnaise is high in fat, so
    should be used sparingly and only occasionally)
2 large lettuce leaves, cut in half
1 dill pickle, thinly sliced (pickles are high in sodium
    and also should be used sparingly)
4 thinly sliced red onion rings

Cut the tempeh in ½-inch-thick slices. Heat the oil in a frying pan and fry the tempeh on both sides until golden brown. Mix the water with the soy sauce, pour over the tempeh, and cook over high heat until all the liquid has evaporated. Spread the bread with the mustard or mayonnaise, or both, and arrange the lettuce on top. Place the fried tempeh on the lettuce and garnish with sliced pickles and onion rings.

Tempeh with Sauerkraut

1 tablespoon corn oil
1 8-ounce block tempeh, cubed
½ medium cabbage, finely sliced
½ cup sauerkraut
1 cup water or sauerkraut juice
½ teaspoon light miso, creamed in 1 tablespoon water
¼ cup finely sliced scallions

Heat the oil in a frying pan and brown the tempeh evenly. Add the cabbage and sauté with the tempeh for 5 minutes. Place the sauerkraut on top, add the water or sauerkraut juice, and steam for 20 minutes. Stir in the dissolved miso and simmer for 5 minutes. Mix in the scallions gently.

Serves 4

Miso Soup

¼ cup dry wakame sea vegetable
4 to 6 cups water
1 medium carrot, cut into matchstick-sized pieces
1 cup thinly sliced white cabbage
½ cup thinly sliced onions
2 to 3 tablespoons miso

Wash the wakame briefly under cold running water to remove dirt and excess salt. Soak for 3 to 5 minutes or until soft and cut into bite-sized pieces. (You may use the soaking water for soup.) Bring the water and wakame to a boil in a saucepan, cover, and simmer over medium-low heat for 8 to 10 minutes. While the wakame is cooking, wash and cut the vegetables. Add them to the saucepan, return to a boil, and simmer over medium-low heat for 8 minutes. Purée the miso with ¼ cup soup water, stir gently to mix with the soup, and simmer over low heat for 3 minutes. Garnish with fresh sliced scallions.

Serves 6

Variation
Use any 3 vegetables of varied color and shape.

Seaweeds

Arame with Lemon Rind and Sesame Seeds

Enjoy this recipe as a vegetable dish or a delicious addition to your favorite salads.

> 1 package (1.7 ounces) arame sea vegetable
> Water
> 1 tablespoon soy sauce
> 1 teaspoon grated lemon rind
> ½ cup ground roasted sesame seeds

Rinse the arame in a strainer under running water. Place the arame in a pot with enough water to cover and let sit for 3 to 5 minutes. Bring to a boil, cover, reduce the heat to medium-low, and simmer for 10 minutes. Remove the lid, add the soy sauce, and boil until all the liquid has evaporated. Add the lemon rind and sesame seeds and mix well. Serve with lemon wedges and garnish with fresh sliced scallions.

Serves 4 to 6

Dulse

Dulse can also be roasted and ground and used as a condiment over grains and vegetables. Dry-roasted dulse makes a tasty addition to sandwiches.

> 1 cup dry dulse
> 2 cups water

Clean the dulse thoroughly by pulling it apart and rinsing well under running water. You may find tiny little shells and pockets of salt hidden away. Soak the dulse in the water for 5 to 15 minutes. Remove it from the soaking water, gently squeeze out the excess liquid, and chop into bite-sized pieces. Add to salads and soups.

Animal Foods
Broiled Fish

1 pound white firm-fleshed fish
½ cup water
¼ teaspoon soy sauce
½ teaspoon ginger juice

Wash the fish quickly under cold running water. Combine the remaining ingredients and soak the fish in the marinade for 1 hour. Place the fish on an oiled baking sheet under the broiler and broil on each side for approximately 5 to 8 minutes. Broiling time depends on the size and thickness of the fish.
  Serves 2 to 4

Variation
Instead of marinating the fish, sprinkle it with lemon juice and a few drops of soy sauce. Serve with lemon wedges, parsley sprigs, or grated raw daikon.

Fish Soup

½ to ¾ pound firm-fleshed fish fillet
1 cup bite-sized pieces collard greens
2 cups thinly sliced leeks (including tops)
1 cup bite-sized pieces Chinese cabbage
6 to 8 cups water
1 stalk kombu, soaked and cut into thin strips
1 pinch salt (optional)
A few drops soy sauce
¼ teaspoon freshly grated ginger

Rinse the fish quickly under cold running water and cut into small pieces. Wash and cut the vegetables as described above. Bring the water and kombu to a boil in a saucepan, add the fish (and salt), cover, and simmer over low heat for 25 minutes.

Add the vegetables, return to a boil, and simmer over low heat for 5 minutes. Season with soy sauce and grated ginger and simmer for 2 minutes. Stir with a wooden spoon to mix the vegetables and fish evenly. Garnish with chopped parsley.

Serves 6

Chicken Soup

1 chicken breast
8 to 10 cups water
1 bay leaf
½ teaspoon oregano
1 teaspoon basil
1 pinch salt
2 medium carrots
2 stalks celery
2 medium onions
1 cup small noodles (elbows, thin spaghetti, alphabets, etc.)
¼ cup chopped parsley
Dash black or white pepper
1 teaspoon soy sauce

Wash the chicken briefly under cold running water. Place the water, chicken, bay leaf, oregano, basil, and salt in a large pot. Bring to a boil, cover, and simmer over medium-low heat for 45 minutes or until the chicken is soft. While the chicken is cooking, wash and dice the carrots and celery and peel and dice the onions. Add them to the chicken broth, return to a boil, and simmer over medium-low heat for 15 minutes. Remove the chicken, debone it, and cut into bite-sized pieces. Skim the chicken fat off the top of the soup. Add the noodles and cook until soft—approximately 5 to 8 minutes. Add the chicken pieces, parsley, pepper, and soy sauce to the soup, return to a boil, and remove from the heat.

Serves 6 to 8

Condiments and Dressings
Sesame Seed Condiment

Sprinkle this condiment over grains or vegetables.

>   10 parts sesame seeds
>   1 part wakame sea vegetable

Wash the sesame seeds thoroughly in a strainer and let stand 5 minutes to drain any remaining water. Place the sesame seeds in a heated skillet and dry roast over low heat. Stir constantly with a wooden spoon, shaking the skillet from time to time so that the seeds roast evenly. When they give off a nutty fragrance, darken in color, and begin to pop (usually within 5 minutes, depending on the amount of seeds used), they are done. Test by crushing a few seeds between thumb and index finger. If they crush easily they are properly done. Remove the seeds from the skillet immediately to prevent burning.

Place the wakame on a cookie sheet. Roast in a 300°F oven for 15 minutes or until crisp. Partially crush the wakame in a blender, mortar and pestle, or suribachi. Add the roasted sesame seeds and grind together until the seeds and seaweed form a coarse powder. Store in a tightly covered jar.

Variation
Substitute dulse or kombu or small dried fish (such as dried sardines) for wakame.

Oil, Vinegar, and Soy Sauce Dressing

>   1 tablespoon brown rice vinegar
>   1 ½ teaspoons sesame, olive, or corn oil
>   ½ teaspoon soy sauce

Do not premix the dressing. Prepare the salad, add the ingredients directly to it, and toss. Serve immediately.

Serves 4 to 6

Scallion-Parsley Dressing

¼ cup finely sliced scallions
1 tablespoon finely chopped parsley
1 teaspoon olive, sesame, or corn oil
1 tablespoon lemon juice
1 tablespoon brown rice vinegar
1 pinch salt
½ cup water

Place all the ingredients in a jar, cover tightly, and shake well.
Pour over a favorite salad, toss, and serve immediately.
    Serves 6

Creamy Tofu Dressing

This dressing is also delicious over noodles.

½ block (8 ounces) soft tofu, drained
¼ small onion, diced
1 tablespoon olive, sesame, or corn oil
2 tablespoons water
1 teaspoon soy sauce

Cream all the ingredients in a suribachi or blender. Pour over a
favorite salad, toss gently, and serve immediately.
    Serves 6

Variation

Tofu Dip or Spread: Substitute chives or scallions for onions.
If you cream the ingredients in a blender, add the chives or
scallions after blending. Serve as a dip with raw vegetables or
salt-free chips or spread on bread or crackers.

Orange Miso Dressing

This dressing is best over leafy green salads.

    1 to 1 ½ teaspoons white miso
    ¼ cup freshly squeezed orange juice
    1 tablespoon ground roasted sesame seeds (optional)

Cream the miso with the orange juice in a suribachi or small bowl. Mix in the sesame seeds and pour over your favorite salad. Toss gently and serve immediately.
    Serves 4

Fruits and Desserts
Gelatin Kanten

A good warm-weather dessert.

    1 quart apple or any other unsweetened fruit juice
    2 tablespoons maple syrup (optional)
    1 pinch salt
    ½ teaspoon vanilla (optional)
    ⅓ cup agar flakes
    1 tablespoon arrowroot or kuzu, dissolved in ¼ cup
      apple juice
    1 tablespoon lemon juice
    1 pint strawberries, washed and quartered

Combine the apple juice, maple syrup, salt, vanilla, and agar flakes in a saucepan and bring to a boil, stirring constantly. Whisk in the arrowroot or kuzu mixture and continue stirring until the mixture returns to a boil. Reduce the heat to medium-low and simmer for 5 minutes. Add the lemon juice. Rinse a square glass pan or bowl with cold water, place the strawberries in the pan, and pour the hot apple juice mixture over the fruit. Chill in the refrigerator until set—

approximately 1 hour. Garnish with chopped nuts and top with Whipped Tofu Cream (see recipe at end of this section).

Serves 4 to 5

Variations

Use thin orange slices (with peel), blueberries, raspberries, mixed soft fruit pieces (watermelon, grapes, peaches, cherries, etc.) instead of strawberries.

To make a creamy pudding, purée the gelatin in a blender, return it to the pan, and chill for 30 minutes.

Coffee Gelatin

4 cups apple juice
2½ tablespoons grain coffee substitute (e.g., Pero, Cafix)
⅓ cup agar flakes
2 tablespoons tahini
¼ teaspoon cinnamon
⅛ teaspoon salt

Whip all the ingredients in a blender. Bring to a boil in a saucepan, reduce the heat to medium-low, and simmer for 5 minutes. Rinse a bowl with cold water, add the hot apple juice mixture, and chill in the refrigerator until set — approximately 1 hour. Garnish with toasted chopped nuts and top with Whipped Tofu Cream (see recipe at end of this section).

Serves 6

Muffins

The sweetener used affects the consistency of these muffins.
Maple syrup produces light ones, while barley malt makes
them moist and heavy.

Dry Ingredients
2 cups pastry flour
1 cup cornmeal
1 tablespoon baking powder (preferably low sodium)
¼ teaspoon cinnamon
⅛ teaspoon salt

Wet Ingredients
¼ to ½ cup maple syrup or ¾ cup barley malt
½ cup corn oil
1 cup water or apple juice
1 teaspoon vanilla (optional)
1 tablespoon orange rind

All the ingredients should be at room temperature. Mix the
dry and wet ingredients separately. Combine both sets of
ingredients in a large bowl and fold gently together — don't
overmix. Preheat the oven to 375°F, oil a muffin tin, and
spoon in the batter until the cups are three-quarters full. Bake
for 20 minutes.

Yields 12 large muffins

Variations

For fruit and nut muffins use blueberries or cranberries,
roasted walnuts, almonds, or sunflower seeds.

For bran muffins use 3 parts flour, 1 part bran, raisins, and
lemon rind.

Substitute soy flour for cornmeal to make lighter muffins.

Blueberry Couscous Cake

This cake takes no oil, flour, or baking.

>   6 cups apple juice
>   2 tablespoons maple syrup (optional)
>   1 teaspoon grated lemon rind
>   1 pinch salt
>   1 teaspoon vanilla
>   2 cups couscous (precooked semolina wheat product)
>   1 pint blueberries, picked over and washed

Bring the apple juice, maple syrup, lemon rind, salt, and vanilla to a boil in a pot. Add the couscous, reduce the heat, and stir until almost thick—approximately 5 minutes. Remove from the heat. Rinse a 9-inch-by-9-inch-square glass baking dish or cake pan with cold water. Arrange the washed blueberries evenly to cover the bottom of the pan. Pour the hot couscous mixture over the blueberries and chill in the refrigerator until set—approximately 45 minutes to 1 hour. Remove from the refrigerator, place a serving platter over the baking dish, and turn it upside down. The cake will slip out easily. Cut into squares. Garnish with chopped toasted nuts and top with Whipped Tofu Cream (see recipe at the end of this section).

    Yields 10 to 15 squares

Variation

Add the blueberries to the hot couscous mixture. Some berries will burst, leaving purple streaks and making the cake very colorful. Strawberries, raspberries, blackberries, or any other soft fruit may be substituted for the blueberries.

Apple Crisp

6 to 8 apples, peeled, cored, and sliced
¼ teaspoon cinnamon
1 cup apple juice
1 cup unbleached white flour
1 cup whole-wheat flour
1 cup rolled oats
1 pinch salt
½ cup chopped roasted walnuts or sunflower seeds (optional)
½ cup corn oil
¼ to ½ cup maple syrup
¼ teaspoon vanilla

Line the bottom of a 9-inch-by-12-inch baking pan with apple slices. Mix the cinnamon with the apple juice and pour over the apples. Mix the flours, oats, salt, and nuts in a bowl. Add the oil, maple syrup, and vanilla and stir until the mixture is crumbly. If it's too dry, add a little apple juice. Sprinkle the crumb mixture over the apples. Bake in a preheated 350°F oven for 40 minutes or until the top begins to brown.
    Serves 6 to 8

Variation
Substitute pears or peaches for apples.

Oatmeal Cookies No. 1

Dry Ingredients
1 cup rolled oats
1½ cups whole-wheat pastry flour
½ teaspoon baking soda
1 teaspoon cinnamon
½ cup chopped roasted walnuts
½ cup raisins (soaked 5 minutes in hot water to cover)

Wet Ingredients
½ cup corn oil
½ cup maple syrup
1 teaspoon vanilla
2 teaspoons rice vinegar

Preheat the oven to 325°F. Mix the dry ingredients, discarding the water in which the raisins were soaked. Blend the wet ingredients. Mix all the ingredients together in a large bowl. Spoon onto an oiled cookie sheet and bake for 15 to 20 minutes.

Yields 24 small cookies

Oatmeal Cookies No. 2

Dry Ingredients
2 cups rolled oats
¾ cup whole-wheat pastry flour
½ cup chopped roasted almonds
½ teaspoon cinnamon
1 pinch salt

Wet Ingredients
¾ cup currants
1 teaspoon grated lemon rind
1 cup apple juice
¼ cup corn oil
2 tablespoons maple syrup

Mix the dry and wet ingredients separately. Combine both sets of ingredients and blend thoroughly. Roll the dough into small balls. Place them on an oiled cookie sheet and press down with a fork. Bake at 350°F until brown — approximately 10 minutes.

Yields 16 cookies

Whipped Tofu Cream

Serve this topping over your favorite desserts or use it as frosting for cakes and cupcakes.

> 1 8-ounce block soft tofu, drained
> ¼ to ½ cup maple syrup
> 1 ½ teaspoons vanilla
> 1 teaspoon grated lemon rind
> 1 teaspoon lemon juice
> 1 pinch salt

Place all the ingredients in a blender and whip for 5 minutes. Turn off the blender and stir with a wooden spoon from the top to the bottom. Whip again for 5 minutes or until completely creamy. Garnish with fresh fruit or roasted nuts.

Serves 4 to 6

Appendix

Fat and Calorie Content of Selected Foods

Beans, Nuts, and Seeds

		% cal/fat	Grams fat	Calories
1 cup	Soybeans, cooked	37	10	234
1 piece	Soybeans, curd (tofu), 2½ × 2¾ × 1″	49	5	86
¼ cup	Peanuts, roasted	70	18	210
¼ cup	Sunflower seeds, hulled	71	17	203
2 Tbsp.	Peanut butter	73	16	188
¼ cup	Almonds, roasted	77	23	246
¼ cup	Walnuts, black, chopped, shelled	79	18	196

Less than 20% calories from fat: Beans (all types except soybeans), bean sprouts, chestnuts, chickpeas.

Reprinted from *Jack Sprat's Legacy: The Science and Politics of Fat and Cholesterol,* which is available from the Center for Science in the Public Interest, 1755 S Street, N.W., Washington, D.C. 20009, for $6.95. Copyright © 1981.

Beef

		% cal/fat	Grams fat	Calories
3 oz.	Beef liver, raw	25	4	150
3 oz.	Round steak, lean only	29	5	161
3 oz.	Sirloin steak, wedge or roundbone, lean only	33	6	176
3 oz.	Flank steak, 100% lean	33	6	167
1 cup	Stewing beef, lean only	40	13	300
3 oz.	Rump roast, lean only	40	8	177
3 oz.	Beef liver, fried	41	9	195
3 oz.	Porterhouse steak, lean only	42	9	190
3 oz.	T-bone steak, lean only	42	9	190
3 oz.	Sirloin steak, hipbone, lean only	47	11	204
3 oz.	Chuck rib roast or steak, lean only	50	12	212
3 oz.	Rib roast, lean only	50	11	205
3 oz.	Round steak, lean w/fat	53	13	222
3 oz.	Ground beef, fairly lean	64	17	235
1 cup	Stewing beef, lean w/fat	66	34	458
3 oz.	Rump roast, lean w/fat	71	23	295

Beef (cont.)

		% cal/fat	Grams fat	Calories
3 oz.	Sirloin steak, wedge or roundbone, lean w/fat	75	27	329
3 oz.	Chuck rib roast or steak, lean w/fat	78	31	363
3 oz.	Rib roast, lean w/fat	81	34	374
3 oz.	Porterhouse steak, lean w/fat	82	36	395
3 oz.	T-bone steak, lean w/fat	82	37	402
3 oz.	Sirloin steak, hipbone, lean w/fat	83	38	414

Breads, Rolls, and Baked Goods

	% cal/fat	Grams fat	Calories
1 med. Doughnut	42	8	164
⅛ commercial ring Danish pastry	49	10	179

Less than 20% of calories from fat: Breads (cracked wheat, French, Italian, white, rye, whole wheat).

Candy

		% cal/fat	Grams fat	Calories
1 oz.	Chocolate, plain	53	9	147

Cereals, Grains, and Pasta

		% cal/fat	Grams fat	Calories
1 Tbsp.	Wheat germ, plain	25	1	23

Note: Granolas contain significant amounts of fat.

Less than 20% of calories from fat: barley, bulgur, macaroni, noodles, oatmeal, rice, spaghetti.

Dairy Products and Eggs

		% cal/fat	Grams fat	Calories
4 oz.	Ice milk, 5.1% fat by weight	29	4	133
1 cup	Milk, 2% w/non-fat solids	30	5	145
8 oz.	Yogurt, low-fat, plain	21	4	144
½ cup	Cheese, cottage	35	4	112
1 cup	Milk, whole	47	8	159
8 oz.	Yogurt, whole milk, plain	48	8	140
4 oz.	Ice cream, reg. (10% fat by weight)	48	7	127
1 oz.	Cheese, mozzarella, part-skim type	55	5	72
½ cup	Cheese, ricotta, part-skim type	50	10	171
1 lg.	Eggs	64	6	82
4 oz.	Ice cream, rich (16% fat by weight)	64	12	165
1 oz.	Cheese, Swiss	66	8	105
½ cup	Cheese, ricotta, whole-milk type	66	16	216

Dairy Products and Eggs (cont.)

		% cal/fat	Grams fat	Calories
1 oz.	Cheese, Cheddar	71	9	113
1 oz.	Cheese, brick	72	9	105
1 oz.	Cheese, Camembert	72	7	85
1 oz.	Cheese, blue or Roquefort	73	9	105
1 Tbsp.	Cream, Half & Half	79	2	20
1 lg.	Egg, yolk	79	5	59
1 Tbsp.	Cream, coffee or light	85	3	32
1 Tbsp.	Cream cheese	90	5	52
1 Tbsp.	Cream, light whipping	92	5	45
1 pat	Butter	100	4	36
1 Tbsp.	Butter	100	12	102

About cheeses: The only hard cheeses with a moderate fat content are the part-skim types. All of the following cheeses are made from whole milk and contain 8 to 9 grams of fat per ounce serving (and at least 60% of the calories from fat): blue, brick, brie, caraway, Cheddar, Edam, Gouda, Gruyère, Limburger, Monterey, Muenster, Port du salut, Provolone, Roman, Roquefort, Swiss; and pasteurized processed American, pimento, and Swiss.

Less than 20% calories from fat: Buttermilk (made from skim milk), uncreamed cottage cheese, skim milk, sherbet, low-fat cottage cheese, uncreamed farmer cheese.

Fish

		% cal/fat	Grams fat	Calories
1 cup	Oysters, raw, meat only	25	4	158
3 oz.	Tuna, chunk, oil-packed, drained very well	37	7	169
3 oz.	Salmon, pink	38	5	120

Fish (cont.)

		% cal/fat	Grams fat	Calories
3 oz.	Salmon, smoked	48	8	150
3 oz.	Salmon, sockeye (red)	49	8	146
3 oz.	Sardines, Atlantic, in oil, 1 can drained	49	9	173
3 oz.	Mackerel, Pacific, canned	50	8	153
5 fillets	Anchovies	54	2	135
3 oz.	Herring, Pacific	59	12	177
3 oz.	Tuna, chunk, oil-packed, undrained	63	17	245

Less than 20% of calories from fat: Cod, crab, flounder, haddock, halibut, lobster, perch, pollock, scallops, sole, shrimp, light tuna in water, some types of albacore tuna in water.

Fruits

		% cal/fat	Grams fat	Calories
½ cup	Coconut, shredded	85	14	138
2 × 2 × ½" piece	Coconut, fresh	85	16	156

Less than 20% calories from fat: Apples, apple butter, apple juice and sauce, apricots, bananas, blackberries, blueberries, boysenberries, sweet cherries, cranberries, cranberry juice cocktail, dates, figs, grapefruits, lemons, lemonade, lychees, mangos, honeydew melons, nectarines, oranges, papayas, peaches, pears, pineapples, plantains, plums, prunes, raisins, raspberries, strawberries, tangerines, watermelons.

Lamb

		% cal/fat	Grams fat	Calories
3 oz.	Leg, lean only	34	6	158
3 oz.	Rib chops, lean only	45	9	180
3 oz.	Leg, lean w/fat	61	16	237
3 oz.	Rib chops, lean w/fat	79	31	355

Pork

		% cal/fat	Grams fat	Calories
3 oz.	Ham, lean only	43	8	159
3 oz.	Boston butt (shoulder), lean only	53	12	207
3 oz.	Ham, lean w/fat	69	19	246
3 oz.	Boston butt (shoulder), lean w/fat	73	24	300
3 oz.	Spareribs	80	33	377
2 med. slices	Bacon	82	8	86

Poultry

Chicken		% cal/fat	Grams fat	Calories
3 oz.	Light meat, w/o skin	23	4	147
3 oz.	Dark meat, w/o skin	43	8	174
3 oz.	Light meat w/skin, roasted	44	9	188
3 oz.	Light meat w/skin, flour-coated and fried	44	10	209

Poultry (cont.)

		% cal/fat	Grams fat	Calories
3 oz.	Light meat w/skin, batter-dipped and fried	50	13	235
3 oz.	Dark meat w/skin, flour-coated and fried	53	14	242
3 oz.	Dark meat w/skin, roasted	56	13	215
3 oz.	Dark meat w/skin, batter-dipped and fried	56	16	253

Turkey

3 oz.	Light meat w/o skin	18	3	133
3 oz.	Dark meat w/o skin	35	6	159
3 oz.	Light meat w/skin	38	7	167
3 oz.	Dark meat w/skin	47	10	188

Other

3 oz.	Goose meat only	48	11	202
3 oz.	Goose meat w/skin	65	19	259
3 oz.	Duck meat only	50	10	171
3 oz.	Duck meat w/skin	76	24	286

Processed Meats

		% cal/fat	Grams fat	Calories
2 oz.	Scrapple	58	8	122
2 oz.	Liverwurst	75	14	174
2 oz.	Salami	76	22	256
2 oz.	Frankfurter	80	16	176
2 slices	Bologna	81	7	80
2 oz.	Country-style sausage	81	18	196
2 oz. (2 links)	Pork sausage	83	11	124

Veal

		% cal/fat	Grams fat	Calories
3 oz.	Round roasts and leg cutlets, lean w/fat	46	9	184
3 oz.	Rib roast, lean w/fat	57	14	229
3 oz.	Breast, lean w/fat	63	18	257

Vegetables

		% cal/fat	Grams fat	Calories
10 med.	French-fried potatoes, 2– 3 ½" long	43	7	137
1 cup	Hash brown potatoes— from frozen	45	18	347
10 chips	Potato chips	62	8	114
½	Avocado	82	19	188
10 small	Olives, green	91	4	33

Bibliography

Chapters 2 and 3

Scientific Papers

"American Dietetic Association Reports: Position Paper on the Vegetarian Approach to Eating." *Journal of the American Dietetic Association* 77 (1980):61.

A thorough and meticulously researched paper in which the ADA reported on the health effects of vegetarian diets (those composed entirely of plant food as well as those which include milk and eggs) and concluded that a diet "consisting of largely unrefined foods" meets all the body's nutrient needs. This is true for both a lacto-ovo vegetarian diet and one composed entirely of plant foods, so long as each is well planned. Furthermore, the ADA recognized the "growing body of scientific evidence" supporting the preventive effects of a vegetarian diet against certain diseases, including cardiovascular disease and cancer.

Blankenhorn, David H., et al. "The Rate of Atherosclerosis Change During Treatment of Hyperlipoproteinemia." *Circulation* 57 (1978):355.

Blankenhorn and his colleagues at the University of Southern California discovered that by using a low-fat, low-cholesterol diet to lower the blood cholesterol of patients with advanced atherosclerosis, the rate of atherosclerosis in the femoral (leg) arteries was markedly reduced.

Gotto, Antonio M. "Is Atherosclerosis Reversible?" *Journal of the American Dietetic Association* 74 (1979):551.

Gotto reviewed the scientific evidence (both human and animal studies) on the effects of diet on atherosclerosis and concluded that, based on the evidence, a low-fat diet does indeed reduce the rate of fat deposits that clog the arteries in humans.

Petrakis, N. L., and King, E. "Cytological Abnormalities in Nipple Aspirates of Breast Fluid from Women with Severe Constipation." *Lancet* 2 (1981):1203.

A report of a study that found a clear correlation between constipation and the rate of abnormalities in breast fluid, breast disease, and mutagenic substances in the intestines.

Sacks, Frank M.; Rosner, Bernard; and Kass, Edward H. "Blood Pressure in Vegetarians." *American Journal of Epidemiology* 100 (1974):5.

A report of a study done by Harvard Medical School scientists who found a correlation between a vegetarian diet (composed of whole grains and vegetables) and lower levels of serum cholesterol.

Shekelle, R. B., et al. "Dietary Vitamin A and Risk of Cancer in the Western Electric Study." *Lancet* 2 (1981):1185.

Researchers correlated the eating and smoking habits of two thousand Western Electric workers and found that those who ate foods rich in the vegetable source of vitamin A (beta carotene), including cigarette smokers, showed the lowest rate of lung cancer.

Stamler, Jeremiah. "Lifestyles, Major Risk Factors, Proof and Public Policy." *Circulation* 58 (1978):3.

One of the best papers available on the abundant evidence linking a high-fat diet to heart and artery diseases, and the need for public policy to reflect this evidence.

Wissler, R. W., and Vesselinovitch, D. "Regression of Atherosclerosis in Experimental Animals and Man." *Modern Concepts of Cardiovascular Disease* 46 (1977):27.

Studies of regression of atherosclerosis in experimental animals and humans indicate that a low-fat, low-cholesterol diet reverses atherosclerotic lesions.

Government Reports and Scientific Testimony before the U.S. Senate

Composition of Foods, Agriculture Handbook No. 8, ed. 8–1 through 8–7. U.S. Department of Agriculture, revised 1976 through 1982.

Available from the Government Printing Office, Washington, DC 20402.

A thorough presentation of the nutritive value of foods.

Diet, Nutrition, and Cancer. The National Research Council of the National Academy of Sciences, 1982. Available from the National Academy Press, 2101 Constitution Avenue, N.W., Washington, DC 20418.

The most thorough and exhaustive presentation of the evidence linking diet to cancer. The 500-page NRC document discusses all the important studies, with footnotes and references, and the council's evaluation of the studies. The NRC also provides dietary guidelines based on the evidence that will probably reduce the risk of cancer.

Dietary Goals for the United States. U.S. Senate Select Committee on Nutrition and Human Needs, 2d ed., December 1977. Available from the Government Printing Office, Washington, DC 20402. Stock No. 052–070–04376–8.

The landmark document that started Americans thinking about their diets, *Dietary Goals* provides dietary recommendations and an overview of the evidence linking diet to disease. The report also provides the results of research on the dietary habits of Americans.

Dietary Guidelines for Americans. U.S. Departments of Agriculture and Health and Human Services, 1980. Available from the Office of Government and Public Affairs, Publication Division, USDA, Washington, DC 20250.

General dietary guidelines similar to those of *Dietary Goals* and *Healthy People.*

Healthy People: The Surgeon General's Report on Health Promotion and Disease Prevention. The U.S. Surgeon General's Office, U.S. Department of Health and Human Services, 1979. Available from the Government Printing Office, Washington, DC 20402. Stock No. 017–001–00416–2.

Provides dietary recommendations and an overview of the evidence linking diet to illness, including cancer and cardiovascular disease.

U.S. Senate Subcommittee on Nutrition. *Heart Disease: Public Health Enemy No. 1* (May 22, 1979). Available from the Government Printing Office, Washington, DC 20402.

U.S. Senate Subcommittee on Nutrition. *Diet and Cancer Relationship* (October 2, 1979). Available from the Government Printing Office, Washington, DC 20402.

The prepared statement of Arthur C. Upton, M.D., of the National Institutes of Health and former director of the National Cancer Institute, is particularly noteworthy because it provides a succinct and thoughtful review of the evidence linking diet to cancer, as well as the leading theories on the ways diet may give rise to this disease.

Books

Arasaki, Seibin, and Arasaki, Teruko. *Vegetables from the Sea.* Tokyo: Japan Publications, 1983.

Everything you ever wanted to know about Japanese seaweeds: how they are grown and prepared and their nutritional content.

Ballantine, Rudolph, M.D. *Diet and Nutrition: A Holistic Approach.* Honesdale, Pa.: Himalayan International Institute, 1978.

A thorough guide to nutrition and the body, as well as an introduction to various Eastern philosophical approaches to diet and health.

Brody, Jane. *The New York Times Guide to Personal Health.* New York: Times Books, 1982.

A collection of Brody's articles on health that originally appeared in the *New York Times.* Subjects range from nutrition, to environmental health hazards, to the health of the elderly.

Colbin, Annemarie. *The Book of Whole Meals.* New York: Ballantine Books, 1983.

Perhaps the best book available on natural food cooking, by the founder of the Natural Gourmet Cookery School in New York City.

Esko, Wendy. *Introducing Macrobiotic Cooking.* Tokyo: Japan Publications, 1978.

An introduction to basic whole food cooking.

Guberlet, Muriel Lewin. *Seaweeds at Ebb-Tide.* Seattle: University of Washington Press, 1971.

Hausman, Patricia. *Jack Sprat's Legacy: The Science and Politics of Fat and Cholesterol.* New York: Richard Marek Publishers, 1981. Also available from the Center for Science in the Public Interest, 1755 S St., N.W., Washington, DC 20009.

The best book written on what fat does to the body, and how industry has prevented this country from establishing a sane nutrition policy.

Hillson, C. J. *Seaweeds*. University Park: Keystone Books, Pennsylvania State University, 1977.

Lappé, Frances M. *Diet for a Small Planet*. New York: Ballantine Books, 1971.

The book that touched off a revolution in nutrition and got people to recognize that one need not eat meat to get adequate nutrition and all the protein the body needs. It also pointed out the social and agricultural problems that result from our society's overdependence on meat as a staple food.

A basic introduction to good nutrition and the health benefits of a low-fat whole-grain and vegetable diet.

Madlener, Judith Cooper. *The Seavegetable Book*. New York: Clarkson N. Potter Publishers, 1977.

One of the best books on harvesting and preparing seaweeds. Madlener provides descriptions, habitats, nutrient content, recipes, and other information on seaweeds that grow in coastal waters all over the world.

Martin, Alice A., and Tenenbaum, Frances. *Diet Against Disease*. Boston: Houghton Mifflin Company, 1980.

An introduction to good diet and nutrition based on *Dietary Goals for the United States*. The book includes recipes.

Pritikin, Nathan. *The Pritikin Promise: 28 Days to a Longer, Healthier Life*. New York: Simon & Schuster, 1983.

Periodicals

Cancer Facts and Figures, 1982. New York: American Cancer Society, 1981.

Fernstrom, John D. "How Food Affects Your Brain." *Nutrition Action* (December 1979):5–7. (A publication of the Center for Science in the Public Interest, Washington, D.C.)

Findlay, Steve. "What's Up, Doc? Can Carrots Prevent Cancer? New Evidence Suggests a Link." *Nutrition Action* (February 1982):12–13.

Leviton, Richard. "Things Go Better with Soyburgers." *East-West Journal* (October 1981):25–29.

Liebman, Bonnie F., and Moyer, Greg. "The Case Against Sugar." *Nutrition Action* (December 1980):9–13.

"A Soyfoods Trailblazer Looks Back and Ahead: An Interview with Dr. Clifford Hesseltine, Chief of Fermentation Laboratory at the U.S. Department of Agriculture." *East-West Journal* (October 1981):30–33.

Hesseltine reports on the nutrient content, especially vitamin B_{12}, in tempeh, miso, and other soyfoods.

Chapter 4

Books

de Langre, Jacques. *The First Book of Do-In.* Magalia, Calif.: Happiness Press, 1971.

A short booklet on the practice of acupressure massage, or Do-In, with an explanation of the philosophy behind the practice and photographs explaining how to perform each exercise. Interested readers may write to Happiness Press, 160 Wycliff Way, Magalia, CA 95954, to obtain a copy of the booklet.

Kushi, Michio. *The Book of Do-In: Exercises for Physical and Spiritual Development.* Tokyo: Japan Publications, 1979.

A more complete explanation of the practices of Do-In, and the philosophy behind the exercises.

Morehouse, Laurence E., Ph.D. *Total Fitness in 30 Minutes a Week.* New York: Simon and Schuster, 1975.

A thorough and readable presentation of what exercise does for the body, and how one can become physically fit safely and efficiently.

Zohman, Lenore R., M.D.; Kattus, Albert, M.D.; and Softness, Donald G. *The Cardiologists' Guide to Fitness and Health Through Exercise.* New York: Simon and Schuster, 1979.

An excellent book on exercises for the heart and cardiovascular system.

Periodicals

Reston, James. "Now, About My Operation in Peking," *New York Times,* July 26, 1971.

———. "A View from Shanghai." *New York Times,* August 22, 1971.

Chapter 5

Books

Arehart-Treichel, Joan. *Biotypes: The Critical Link Between Your Personality and Your Health.* New York: Times Books, 1980.
   A thoughtful analysis filled with fascinating case histories, including the Roseto, Pennsylvania, story.
Cousins, Norman. *Anatomy of an Illness as Perceived by the Patient.* New York: W. W. Norton and Company, 1979.
   An inspiring and important account of how one man marshaled his body's immune system to defeat a perilous disease for which medicine had no answer. Cousins also offers a thoughtful analysis of how the mind, particularly its creative faculties, enhances body and brain chemistry and promotes long life.
Dossey, Larry, M.D. *Space, Time and Medicine.* Boulder, Colo.: Shambhala, 1982.
   An excellent presentation of the new physics, and a thorough analysis of how our perceptions of time and state of mind affect our health.
Friedman, Meyer, M.D., and Rosenman, Ray H., M.D. *Type A Behavior and Your Heart.* New York: Alfred A. Knopf, 1974.
   A pioneering work by two cardiologists who showed how stress affects the cardiovascular system and depresses the body's ability to fight disease.
Null, Gary. *Biofeedback, Fasting, and Meditation.* New York: Pyramid Publications, 1974.
   An introduction to meditation and its ability to influence the body.
Peale, Norman Vincent. *The Power of Positive Thinking.* Englewood Cliffs, N.J.: Prentice-Hall, 1952. Long before science validated the power of the mind to influence the physical body and external realities, Peale created a self-help program based on faith and positive thinking. Though written more than thirty years ago, this book still has a great deal to tell us — further evidence of its lasting value.

Simonton, O. Carl, M.D.; Matthews-Simonton, Stephanie; and Creighton, James L. *Getting Well Again*. Los Angeles: J. P. Tarcher, 1978.

The Simontons were among the first researchers to apply the mind-body connection to those with terminal cancer. In the process they helped a surprising number of people overcome their disease and extended the lives of many more. This important pioneering book reports on their experiences, as well as on the evidence linking the mind and body.

Periodicals

Anderson, Alan. "How the Mind Heals." *Psychology Today* (December 1982):51–56.

Wallis, Claudia. "Stress: Can We Cope?" *Time,* June 6, 1983.

Chapter 6

Books

Blakney, R. B., trans. *Tao Te Ching,* Lao-tzu. New York: New American Library, 1955.

The seminal work on one of the most important and widespread religions in the East.

Campbell, Joseph, ed. *The Portable Jung.* New York: Viking Press, 1971.

Fifteen collected works of Carl G. Jung, including his book *Answer to Job.*

Capra, Fritjof. *The Tao of Physics.* Berkeley, Calif.: Shambhala Publications, 1975.

The first book to make quantum mechanics, and so many of its extraordinary discoveries about the nature of the universe, accessible to the nonscientist. Capra went a quantum step further by demonstrating that the new physics offers a view of the universe that is fundamentally analogous to traditional spiritual and religious teachings, particularly those of the East.

Hall, Calvin S., and Nordby, Vernon J. *A Primer of Jungian Psychology.* New York: New American Library, 1973.

An introduction to Jung and his views on the human psyche.

Pagels, Heinz R. *The Cosmic Code: Quantum Physics as the Language of Nature.* New York: Simon and Schuster, 1982.

Quantum mechanics for the nonscientist.

Stevenson, Kenneth E., and Habermas, Gary R. *Verdict on the Shroud: Evidence for the Death and Resurrection of Jesus Christ.* Ann Arbor, Mich.: Servant Books, 1981.

Two former members of the Shroud of Turin research project, the team of scientists who evaluated the burial cloth reputed to be that of Jesus Christ, discuss the findings of the team's research as well as the age-old debate of naturalism versus supernaturalism.

Tillich, Paul. *The Meaning of Health.* Richmond, Calif.: North Atlantic Books, 1981.

In this thorough and enlightening analysis, Tillich discusses the relationship between spiritual growth and physical health.

Wheelwright, Philip, ed. *The Presocratics.* Indianapolis, Ind.: Odyssey Press, 1966.

A review of the early Greek philosophers, from Xenophanes to Hippocrates.

Wolf, Fred Alan. *Taking the Quantum Leap.* New York: Harper and Row, 1981.

A readable and entertaining introduction to the new physics.

Periodicals

Barnhouse, Ruth Tiffany, M.D., Th.M. "Spiritual Direction and Psychotherapy." *Journal of Pastoral Care* 33 (1979):149.

Jack, Alex. "From Science to Society: Fritjof Capra Makes a Quantum Leap." *East-West Journal* (March 1982):28–36.

An interview with Capra.

Chapter 7

Books

Kaplan, Justin. *Walt Whitman: A Life.* New York: Simon and Schuster, 1982.

Moody, Raymond A., Jr., M.D. *Life After Life.* Covington, Ga.: Mockingbird Books, 1975.

Accounts of people who had remarkable experiences during the period called clinical death.

Sabom, Michael B., M.D. *Recollections of Death.* New York: Harper and Row, 1982.

More experiences during clinical death, which, after scientific scrutiny, led to many interesting findings.